FROM HEALTH DOLLARS
TO HEALTH SERVICES

FROM
HEALTH DOLLARS
TO
HEALTH SERVICES
New York City,

1965–1985

ELI GINZBERG
AND THE
CONSERVATION OF HUMAN RESOURCES
STAFF

LandMark Studies
ROWMAN & ALLANHELD
PUBLISHERS

ROWMAN & ALLANHELD
Published in the United States of America in 1986
by Rowman & Allanheld, Publishers
(a division of Littlefield, Adams & Company)
81 Adams Drive, Totowa, New Jersey 07512.

Library of Congress Cataloging-in-Publication Data

Ginzberg, Eli, 1911–
  From health dollars to health services.
  Includes bibliographical references and index.
  1. Medical economics—New York (N.Y.)—History.
2. Medical care—New York (N.Y.)—History. I. Conservation of Human Resources Project (Columbia University) II. Title. [DNLM: 1. Health Services—economics—United States. W 84 AA1 G4f]

RA410.54.N7G56 1986 338.4′73621′097471 85-22309
ISBN 0-8476-7440-1

86 87 88 / 10 9 8 7 6 5 4 3 2 1

Printed in The United States of America

To
Ethel and Marcy Blinken
Friends of Many Years

The Conservation of Human Resources Project

Howard Berliner
Edward A. Brann
Charles Brecher
Victoria Brent
Edith M. Davis
Matthew Drennan
Maury Forman
Michael L. Millman
Dean Morse
Miriam Ostow
Penny Peace
Paul Thompson

Contents

Tables

Foreword

In the writing of books, as in other undertakings, the best laid plans sometimes go awry. This study was planned and much of the initial research was carried out several years ago when, because of conflicting priorities, the draft chapters had to be put aside. In succeeding years, additional investments of staff time and effort were devoted to filling gaps in data and analysis and updating the existing manuscript. However, it was not until the summer of 1983 that I was able to give undivided attention to the study and it was then rewritten in its entirety, except for the last chapter which dates from the summer of 1984.

The basic funding for the study was provided by The Robert Wood Johnson Foundation. The final manuscript, however, has also benefited from the fact that the Conservation of Human Resources Project, Columbia University, has since 1982 received support from The Commonwealth Fund to study the four academic health centers in Manhattan—New York University, Cornell–New York Hospital, Mt. Sinai, and Columbia–Presbyterian. The concluding chapter in particular reflects the synergistic effects of the latter Project.

The extended period of time during which work was under way on the manuscript also explains two facts about the staff: the large number of people who participated in some stage of the research, and the many who are no longer members of the Conservation Project.

I would like to acknowledge the special assistance which we received from various individuals and institutions during the course of our research. They include, in particular: Mrs. Nora Piore, whose pioneering studies of the flow of funds into the health care system in New York City have provided a model for subsequent inquiries; Mr. Cyril Brosnan and the staff of Blue Cross–Blue Shield of Greater New York who made it possible for my associate, Mrs. Miriam Ostow, to select and study in detail the experiences of a sample of twenty-four hospitals during the critical decade following the passage of Medicare and Medicaid; Dr. Joseph English, who first introduced us to the administration of St. Vincent's Hospital and Medical Center, and to Sisters Evelyn Schneider and Margaret Sweeney, its most recent presidents; Mrs. Dorothy Levenson, historian of Montefiore, and our liaison who directed us to the many sources of information within the Medical Center and helped to broaden our understanding of that complex institution; Mr. Stanley Brezenoff who exposed us to the perceptions of City government; the United Hospital Fund of Greater New York; and the New York City Health and Hospitals Corporation.

Dr. Joan M. Leiman generously critiqued the final manuscript. Her comments, observations, and corrections, drawn from long and intimate experience with the New York health care sector and local government, have strengthened the book. Her contribution, however, in no way implies responsibility for its contents and conclusions.

Manuscript preparation that stretches over an extended period of time and involves much writing and rewriting always places an added strain on the secretarial staff. I am particularly grateful for the excellent support I received from Mrs. Sylvia Leef and Ms. Shoshana Vasheetz, who transcribed and kept control over the many drafts of the many chapters.

ELI GINZBERG, Director
Conservation of Human Resources
Columbia University

1

Focus and Themes

High on the national agenda is the question of how to contain the rising costs of medical care. From 1964 to 1984, total outlays in current dollars have increased from approximately $37 billion to $362 billion. The increase is considerably less in constant dollars, but it is still substantial. Even when the constant dollar increases are measured on a per capita basis which reflects the growth of the population, the increase, from $179 to $1,521, is still striking.

Health analysts have broken down this large current dollar increase into a limited number of factors. They ascribe about 60 percent to inflation; less than 10 percent to population increase; and the remainder to "intensity" which reflects real increases in inputs of technology, materials, and human resources but which also includes increased prices for those inputs which have exceeded the average increase in the cost of living index. While these national data provide a framework for assessing broad changes over time, they lump together many discrete patterns of health or medical care that are specific to location, class, or race.

The focus of this inquiry is the impact of the enlarged flow since the mid–1960s of health care dollars on the output of health care services for a discrete population, namely, persons who live in New York City, plus a small but significant number of nonresidents (circa 10 percent) who seek medical, particularly hospital, care in the City. There are several reasons for selecting this focus.

First, it will be possible to trace in considerable detail the process whereby new dollars were transmuted into new or additional services and to pinpoint the principal beneficiaries of this enlarged and improved flow of services. It also will be possible to obtain a first approximation of the critical linkages among additional dollars, more and better services, and improved health outcomes. The last can be gauged by selected criteria of change in health status and/or patient satisfaction as well as broadened access.

The focus of a discrete population in a discrete area facilitates analyzing how the added dollar inflow was channeled among different providers: in the first instance, among physicians, hospitals, nursing homes, and clinics; in the second, among different types of physicians such as office or hospital based, general practitioners, or specialists; as well as among different types of institutions—voluntary and municipal hospitals, skilled nursing homes, and other health-related facilities.

Furthermore, New York City has long been a leading center for medical education and research as well as for medical care delivery, with six (until recently, seven) academic health centers and a number of teaching hospitals of national and international renown. In addition, New York City has financed with public dollars an elaborate municipal hospital system providing both ambulatory and inpatient care to all, regardless of ability to pay. In short, New York City has been committed to taking care of its poor, elderly, and disabled and in fact did so long before the federal government, in 1965, legislated Medicare and Medicaid which radically altered the financing of health care during the two decades under review.

The continuing dynamism of the City—reflected in changes in its total population as well as in its distinct groups; in the disproportionate numbers of persons with low incomes who reside in the City; in the shrinkage in its job base and in particular jobs for the less educated and less skilled; in the influx of large numbers of newcomers from abroad, legal and illegal; in the strength of the trade union movement; in its fiscal crisis in the mid–1970s; in the entrenched role of philanthropy and all the other characteristics and changes in its physical and human resources—provides a rich background against which to investigate and assess the impact of the recent large inflow of health care dollars on the delivery of health services.

So much for focus. A word about the major themes that will be addressed in each of the succeeding chapters. Our plan is to trace seriatim the key steps of the process by which additional health dollars were transformed into additional services and to identify which groups benefited from this stream. In the final two chapters, we will pull these several strands together, look at the transformational process as a whole, and extract the major lessons from that rich experience. This should prove helpful as the nation struggles to improve its health care policy at every level—local, state, and federal.

The principal aim of Chapter 2 is to present an overview of health delivery in New York City in sufficient detail so that the reader can appreciate the magnitude of the sums that flowed into the health care sector in the City between the early 1960s, prior to the passage of Medicare and Medicaid, and 1984. These data will provide information not only about the total inflow in selected years but also about the major sources of funding, particularly the relative shares of the public and private sectors, and within the public sector, the relative importance of federal, state, and local government. Chapter 2 will also identify the principal recipients of these increased funds noting in particular the additional revenues garnered by hospitals, nursing homes, and physicians, which together were the chief beneficiaries of the enlarged resources.

In Chapter 3 we look at the changes that took place in the number of beds, services, and other critical activities during the years when hospitals received many of the new financial resources. Most of the increases took place during the decade 1965–1975 because thereafter the State of New York determined the reimbursement rates of hospitals with respect to their Blue Cross and Medicaid patients. Together, these two categories in 1982 accounted for 44.6 percent of all patient days, exceeding the 40 percent figure that represented Medicare's share of the inpatient total. Chapter 3 leaves no doubt that most hospitals responded aggressively in the late 1960s and early 1970s to the availability of new funding by broadening and deepening their range of services to inpatients and to ambulatory patients as well.

The principal theme of Chapter 3 is to explore the multiple adaptations the hospitals made once they obtained ready access to a new flow of dollars. For a time, they were able to spend first and expect to be reimbursed later with little risk that the payers would not honor their documented expenditures. It was only after the State of New York tightened its controls over Blue Cross and Medicaid reimbursements that the hospitals understood that the sky was not the limit and that they could not assume that their expenditures would be repaid in full.

Prior to the increased availability of funds from Medicare and Medicaid, voluntary hospitals had to consider carefully which of the new diagnostic or therapeutic advances they most wanted or needed. The more powerful chiefs of services in the major teaching hospitals lobbied with each other, with the administrator, and even with the trustees for their preferences, explaining that unless their budgets were increased they could no longer remain at the frontiers of medicine and the hospital would lose its position of prominence. Some of the more aggressive chiefs were able to persuade wealthy patients to make large donations so that the hospital could obtain the new technology and sometimes the gift was ample enough to pay for the additional staff. From time to time, hospitals embarked upon a fund

raising campaign. In a few favored institutions, a wealthy and dedi-
cated board of directors would dig into its own pocket and approach
wealthy associates for contributions.

The only other significant funding sources were research grants
from the National Institutes of Health and the pharmaceutical companies and grants from the federal-state Hill-Burton program for
construction. But in both instances, even strong institutions had to
compete for new resources.

Prior to the establishment of Medicare and Medicaid, hospitals had
to raise the philanthropic funds needed to purchase new equipment
and they also had to consider whether the new equipment would
require additional staff and how much that new staff would cost. Since
labor costs account for about 60 percent of total hospital costs, this
consideration acted as a further constraint on how fast even financially well-situated institutions could add new, expensive equipment.
Although patients covered by commercial insurance or Blue Cross,
together with a few wealthy self-paying patients, would not be de-
terred by rapidly rising per diem costs, hospitals kept tight control on
their expenditures because they recognized that the other 60 or so
percent of their patient flow would be price-sensitive.

After Medicare and Medicaid were enacted, hospitals could look
forward to reimbursement of their costs by third parties not for 40 percent but for 80 percent and eventually over 90 percent of their
total inpatient population. They were in a new world in which they no
longer had to deliberate about whether they could afford large new
expenditures. They could follow an aggressive investment policy, se-
cure in the knowledge that their additional costs would be covered by
third-party reimbursers.

The first six years of the decade after the introduction of Medicare
and Medicaid, between 1966 and 1972, were the golden age for
hospital financing. Hospitals could spend as much as they wanted with
reasonable assurance that they would be reimbursed. In fact, in the
first two years after Medicare was legislated, the law provided for a
2 percent override to hospitals of the costs of treating the beneficiaries
for whom the federal government was responsible. The new reimbursement policy led to a marked upgrading of acute care hospitals
under voluntary auspices.

In Chapter 4 the analysis shifts from a macro view of the acute
hospitals as a group to a micro consideration of two long-established
institutions, St. Vincent's in lower Manhattan and Montefiore in the
west Bronx, the former closely aligned with the Archdiocese of New
York City, the latter with the Federation of Jewish Philanthropies. The
critical question that is explored is the way in which these two institutions took advantage of the new inflow of dollars to transform them-

selves from relatively modest hospitals into major medical centers with greatly enlarged competences.

Prior to the new legislation, the only prospect for such substantial transformations to occur at both St. Vincent's and Montefiore would have been long-term efforts to raise many millions of philanthropic dollars. But the substantially increased flow of public funds, primarily from Medicare and Medicaid but also from other federal, state, and even local sources, created new opportunities for boards, administrators, and staffs not mired in tradition.

The different strategy followed by each institution in its transformation into a comprehensive medical center is reviewed and attention is directed to the challenges that each encountered as it expanded its vision and goals while retaining and even strengthening its ability to continue operating as a voluntary institution. Each was determined, despite its aggressive pursuit of public funds, to continue to operate under an independent board of trustees, with roots in the nongovernmental sector, committed to realizing a number of different goals— medical, educational, social, religious.

The term "entrepreneur" is usually reserved for a businessman operating in competitive markets in pursuit of profits. A close reading of the transformational dynamics of Montefiore Hospital, however, reveals that the term can as readily be applied to the chief official of the hospital who over the years developed the vision and, under a broad grant of authority from his trustees, was responsible for turning his vision into reality. His talent and achievement as a public entrepreneur was not that he sought or made profits, but that he demonstrated unique skill in acquiring the substantial resources to transform his institution from a modest hospital into a leading medical center.

In Chapter 5 the central question considered is the effect of the large new inflow of funds on the municipal hospital system which, prior to the introduction of Medicare and Medicaid, had provided essential medical care for most of the poor and many of the near-poor in several arenas, inpatient, ambulatory, and, to a limited degree, chronic care. A principal objective of the new federal legislation was to move the country toward a single level of care by entitling the elderly and the poor (and after 1972 the permanently disabled as well) to obtain services from any provider. In light of the much older and more developed system of care for the indigent in New York City, we might have expected that the movement towards a single level of care would have been accelerated but the record suggests otherwise.

In 1961, several years before the introduction of Medicare and Medicaid, the City found it necessary to enter into "affiliation contracts" with the large voluntary teaching hospitals to assure adequate professional staffing for its municipal hospitals. Many municipal hospitals were no longer able to attract, as they had in prior decades, the number and range of physicians and specialists required to staff their inpatient and ambulatory services. Their best prospect of meeting their responsibilities to the public was to enter into a contract with a leading teaching hospital. In addition to the dollar payments they received for assigning staff, the contracting institutions welcomed the opportunity to expand their residency training programs. While the affiliation contracts helped to solve the problem of staffing the municipal hospitals, it left open the challenge of balancing the goals of the teaching hospitals with their emphasis on specialized training and the needs of the City whose primary concern was providing essential care to the indigent.

Further complications arose from the partial realization of the federal objective to move the health care system closer to providing a single level of care. After Medicare was established, many of the elderly were able to seek private care and a considerable number of Medicaid patients, especially in the early years, likewise shifted from municipal to voluntary hospitals for ambulatory and inpatient care. Both moves had a depressing effect on the work load of the municipal system.

As Chapter 7 details, the new flows of dollars into the health care system provided the basis for sizable increases in the wages and benefits of all hospital workers in both the municipal and voluntary systems. Although efforts had been made in the pre–1965 years to improve the wages and working conditions of hospital workers which had lagged behind the rest of the economy, the improved flow of funding that followed speeded the process of improvement. The rapid progress of unionization of hospital workers further accelerated their gains.

Prior to the passage of Medicare and Medicaid, the City had tight control over its total dollar expenditures for health care for the indigent. Medicare and Medicaid, however, stripped the City of such fiscal control by "entitling" patients to care and at the same time authorizing them to seek treatment from providers of their choice. Decision-making about which persons would be covered and the range of services to which they would be entitled shifted to the federal and state governments. To complicate matters, the City of New York was obligated to cover 25 percent of all Medicaid costs. With eligibility determined by higher levels of government, with patients free to choose providers, and with the City obligated to meet 25 percent of rising Medicaid costs, the previously controlled commitment of municipal government for health care for the indigent was cut loose from its budgetary moorings with the consequence that the cost to the City in tax-levied dollars (paid for by taxpayers in the City) increased rapidly.

Municipal government encountered additional financial pressures from: the rapidly rising costs of the affiliation contracts; the steep increases in its hospital wage bill; its loss of many patients who sought hospitalization in the voluntary system; the increasing number of uninsured patients who sought treatment; and the difficulties that the new administrative structure—the New York City Health and Hospitals Corporation established in 1970—experienced in billing for reimbursement.

One aspect of the changing role of physicians in the health care system of New York City (Chapter 6) was the difficulty encountered by the municipal hospital system after World War II in attracting medical staff for inpatient and ambulatory care services. The reasons reflected diverse developments, including the relocation to the suburbs of large numbers of middle-class white families which was the prelude to the relocation of many medical practitioners, and the disinclination of newly licensed physicians to open practices in neighborhoods heavily populated by minority poor who had replaced relocating whites.

A second development was an accelerated shift to specialization. This resulted in a steep decline during the 1960s and 1970s in the absolute and relative numbers of general practitioners able and willing to provide primary care services to low-income families. Physicians, particularly the younger trained specialists, were able to build lucrative practices among middle-class and affluent clienteles. They shunned a volume practice at low unit fees which had long been the pattern among many physicians who had previously practiced in low-income neighborhoods.

A related change, speeded by the declining number of primary care physicians in private practice, was the growing tendency of the poor and the near-poor to seek ambulatory care from the outpatient departments and emergency rooms of municipal and voluntary hospitals located in their immediate or nearby neighborhoods. The marked expansion of residency and fellowship training conducted by teaching hospitals, particularly those serving as the principal hospital of an academic health center, provided large house staffs that could be drawn on to provide care in the burgeoning hospital ambulatory services.

The other striking development of the post–World War II era was the large and growing proportion of all licensed physicians who were foreign medical graduates (FMGs). The less prestigious the hospital, the less strong its residency programs, the more it had to rely on filling its residencies with FMGs, most of whom succeeded in acquiring U.S. citizenship during or after completing their training.

Since our basic focus is on the interaction between money flows and the adaptations of the health care system, the following should be emphasized: the ability of hospitals to obtain reimbursement for the escalating salaries they paid residents and the costs of training them by including these expenditures in their per diem costs which third parties were willing to cover. Furthermore, third-party payers were increasingly willing to provide reimbursement for beneficiaries of expanded insurance policies who used emergency rooms and in some cases outpatient departments. Many teaching hospitals, especially those located in low-income neighborhoods, complained about the large numbers of ambulatory patients whom they treated who were not covered by any payer. This led both Blue Cross and the State of New York to allocate special sums to help these institutions cover part of these expenditures.

In Chapter 7 we also address in some detail the question of how the much larger inflow of funds into the health care system altered the status and earnings of the nonprofessional employees who worked in municipal or voluntary hospitals. First, we must recall that before the new health legislation, workers were poorly recompensed, earning considerably below the average of comparable workers in other industries even allowing for the fact that they frequently received free meals or were cared for by the institution and its staff if they became ill. Furthermore, many were not closely supervised which meant that they could get through their daily routine without much effort. These minor advantages aside, however, hospital workers on the lower end of the scale had poor jobs which offered little compensation and few career opportunities.

Hospital administrators admitted that they paid low salaries to persons hired to keep the institution clean, to serve meals, and to carry out other unskilled tasks. They justified their wage scales by pointing to the large numbers of applicants who sought this kind of employment and to the fact that both the municipal and the voluntary hospitals operated under constrained fiscal conditions. These hospitals had to extract their operating funds from tight-fisted legislators or rely on philanthropy to meet their deficits.

As we have seen, the initial impact of Medicaid was to provide the City of New York with a new flow of funds from the federal and state governments amounting to 75 percent of the costs of treating the newly entitled population. And the elderly poor, many of whom had previously sought and received treatment free of charge in municipal hospitals, were soon able to have most, if not all, of their care paid for by Medicare. Additional federal money from categorical and other types of health programs became available in the middle and late

1960s; this set the stage for a vast improvement in the economic position of hospital workers.

With regard to the work force in the municipal hospitals, Mayor John V. Lindsay recognized the justice and the logic of the claims of the workers at the bottom of the ladder for significant increases in their wages and fringe benefits. These claims were pursued by nascent trade unions under aggressive leadership and reinforced by additional pressure from the Civil Rights movement which sought to help the many black hospital workers. Finally, those who held political office and who looked forward to a long-term political career saw significant gains from developing a large new constituent group of better paid unionized workers.

For many years the voluntary hospitals had followed a tight-fisted policy in setting wages for their nonprofessional personnel. But Medicare and Medicaid reduced resistance to a better wage scale. After all, for the first time hospitals were able to recapture from third-party payers all legitimate costs incurred in providing care to the patients they treated. Hospital administrators knew that they were paying their unskilled staff less than what comparable workers earned in the private sector and now that their financial integrity appeared to be assured, they were more willing to raise their wage structure. Moreover, the significant gains achieved by municipal hospital workers added to the willingness of the voluntary sector to adjust wage scales.

The new sources of hospital revenue resulted not only in a significant upward revision of the wage scale and the fringe benefits of hospital workers but also in a substantial addition in the number of workers. In part, these increases reflected downward adjustments in work schedules; in part, they were brought about by the concurrent movement toward more intensive forms of therapy which required that hospitals hire more clinical and support personnel. One of the most important and lasting consequences of the new money flows into the health care system was the qualitative transformation of hospital employment from low paying, unattractive jobs without fringe benefits and little union protection to much better paying jobs with good benefits and strong unions and with at least modest opportunities for career advancement. And these jobs became available to blacks and other minorities at a time when blue-collar employment opportunities in the City were shrinking.

Chapter 8 provides a summary assessment of the achievements made possible through the new financing, a fragile assessment since all societal reforms are likely to achieve only part of their goals. For instance, Medicare surely contributed significantly to improving the access of the elderly to both inpatient and ambulatory care and went a fair distance to fulfilling the implicit and explicit hope that the new legislation would move the country toward a single standard of health care delivery. And it is true that Medicaid also made a modest contribution to help the poor toward that same end.

On the other hand, the growing dependence of the poor and even the elderly on ambulatory care from the outpatient departments of neighborhood hospitals or from the new Medicaid mills which opened up throughout the City has not been a step toward the goal of a single level of care.

Nevertheless, it would be an error to relate these failures solely to the additional dollar flows. They were closely tied to the major demographic shifts which transformed the City and turned many neighborhoods from white middle-class environments to black and Puerto Rican enclaves of low-income families.

When the new health legislation was first passed, many friendly as well as unfriendly critics feared that with the dollar barrier removed, the demand for health care services would skyrocket to a point where all providers would be swamped. That did not happen. But what was not anticipated and did occur was the steep and continuing acceleration of health care costs which led the authorities in Albany to step in and regulate, with increasing stringency, the rates that hospitals could charge third-party payers, specifically Medicaid and Blue Cross. Although there may be some disagreement about the responsibility of these tight reimbursement controls by the State of New York for the deterioration of the hospital plant throughout the state, most experts agree that cost containment in New York State was surely a contributory factor.

Another unexpected consequence was an increased number of nursing homes, largely under private ownership and greatly stimulated by the introduction of Medicaid. Nursing home care currently accounts for about 35 percent of all Medicaid outlays in the state.

Prior to the 1965 legislation, the poor and the near-poor in New York City had been cared for by a combination of municipal funds largely supporting the system of public hospitals and clinics, and the sizable contribution that many voluntary hospitals made to provide ambulatory and inpatient care free of charge or below cost to the near-poor and the poor. In both systems, established physicians as well as residents, were accustomed to donating regularly a great many hours for modest or no pay. We have noted that in the municipal system this critical professional resource had begun to dry up by the early 1960s but voluntary hospitals were still able to draw on a great amount of free service in return for which physicians obtained valuable training, some eventually receiving staff privileges.

The new infusion of government money brought a speedy end to this long-established pattern of free labor. Thereafter, every service which a physician performed would be paid for by somebody, the patient, an insurance plan, or the government. The long-term monetarization of the health care system has never been submitted to the detailed analysis it justifies, but even without such an analysis we can state that the process of monetarization contributed to the escalation of health care costs.

Altering the financial base of a major service delivery system such as health care was certain to have consequences that even the most careful planners could not foresee. But in the case of Medicaid there had been little if any planning. Moreover, potent as money is in shaping the behavior of persons seeking care as well as those providing care, alterations in the money stream never occur in isolation; there are always other significant changes—demographic, institutional, political. The new dollars that flowed into the health care system resulted in many changes some of which were sought, others that had not been anticipated.

The last two decades have witnessed significant changes in the health care delivery system across many fronts—from the new goals of access and equity to increasing the inflow of financial and other resources needed to undergird hospital finances. Since we will have assessed in earlier chapters the interplay among goals, resources, and accomplishments, we draw up a balance sheet in Chapter 9 and seek to extract the principal lessons embedded in our recent experience in the hope of using them as a guide to policy-making in the years ahead. And finally Chapter 10, drawing on all that has gone before, seeks direction for the future.

The only certainty in the highly uncertain arena of health care is the continuing need at every level—national, state, and local—to monitor the level and quality of care provided to all members of the population, to explore the alternative means of raising the resources required to provide the desired level of services, and to work towards a balanced system of incentives and constraints to contribute to the more effective utilization of the available resources.

What can the review of the New York City story contribute to these challenges that continue to confront the health care system?

First, the new dollars that resulted from the passage of Titles XVIII and XIX of the Social Security Act (Medicare and Medicaid) in 1965 were aimed at improving the access of the elderly and the poor to the system. While we have no baseline evaluation of the ease or difficulty that these two major groups faced in 1965 in obtaining access to a broad range of services in New York City, we will not be far off the mark if we reconstruct the situation as follows: the elderly and the poor in New York City were better off than in most other metro-

politan centers because of the sizable municipal hospital system and
the substantial contributions of the voluntary sector to their care.
Nevertheless, a gap existed between resources and demand or need.
In 1982, Louis Harris undertook a major poll for The Commonwealth
Fund which revealed that only a small minority, some 160,000 individuals out of a population of about 7.1 million, or under 2.5 percent,
reported that they had been unable to obtain medical care during the
course of the year. The overwhelming majority, about eight or nine in
every ten persons, reported that they were satisfied with the care that
they and their children obtained. Of course, the public's satisfaction
with the medical care it receives is not the only criterion. The judgment of professionals about the amount and quality of care that
people receive is also important and their judgment would probably
be somewhat less favorable.

A balance sheet would also have to take account of the newly
broadened options of the elderly who now can seek care in the
voluntary sector, the expanded opportunities for the poor to be
treated by private practitioners or in community clinics, and their
much expanded access to nursing homes and home health care—all of
which represent significant gains. It should be clear that much of the
new money was transmuted into more and better health care for the
principal targeted groups.

Our remaining challenge is to call attention to the selected lessons
that can be extracted from the experiences of these tumultuous years.
Despite the large increase in the total dollars that flowed into the
system, approximately sevenfold uncorrected for inflation and population change and about threefold in constant dollars per capita,
severe financial pressures can still be identified: delayed maintenance
and renovation of hospital plants; inadequate staffing in most municipal hospitals and in some voluntary hospitals; the burden on elderly
persons who require costly drugs to control chronic illnesses; the high
costs to middle-class families of maintaining the disabled elderly at
home or providing suitable nursing home care for them; the big bite
that steadily rising insurance costs are taking out of the wage/benefit
packages of many workers; the dire consequences to the minority
without broad insurance coverage who encounter major illness.

The only reasonable conclusion from this summary review of dollar
flows is that in an expanding arena such as health care, where new
knowledge and new technology keep pushing at the frontiers, there
will always be a sizable gap between dollars available and services
wanted and needed. As earlier shortcomings are corrected, new deficiencies are recognized. The real challenge to public policy therefore
must always extend beyond the important issue of funding. The
public must continue to debate and decide upon new goals, new

priorities, and new methods aimed at improved utilization. Dollars alone can never provide the answer. This is the most important lesson that emerges from the New York City story.

In addition, the major institutions that are in place at the time new resources become available are in the best position to capture a share and to use them to further their own goals which may be only loosely linked to the goals of the program. The academic health centers, nonprofessional hospital employees, office- and hospital-based physicians all enjoyed sizable gains as a result of the new dollar influx. While one could establish ties between these gains and improved access to health care services for the elderly and the poor, the linkages are weak.

Another important lesson to be extracted from the New York City story relates to the ebb and flow of political support for public programs. When Medicaid was first introduced, the New York State legislature entitled about one-third of the State's population. Within two years, it retreated and since then has been trimming at the edges, and in periods of financial difficulty has cut into the heart of the program. Since major reforms always require a long period of time for existing institutions to adapt and for new ones to be established, the relatively brief spurts of enthusiasm that capture the political leadership and the public are seldom adequate to assure the restructuring of a complex social system.

Partly for the reasons already mentioned and partly because the full range of consequences of new programs, even with careful planning, cannot be foreseen, it is important to introduce significant innovations in a measured way so that opportunity is offered for all the concerned parties to make adjustments which do not undermine their long-term capacity to perform. The unexpected and rapid acceleration of health care costs following the introduction of Medicare and Medicaid had such untoward consequences that the State of New York found it necessary to intervene in the reimbursement process by setting ceilings which in turn went far to destabilize the hospital's capital plant.

In contrast to the belief of some enthusiasts, the delivery of health care cannot be left to the market alone. Large amounts of new money are usually required to accomplish worthwhile societal objectives. The New York City story should, however, serve as a reminder and a warning that significant reforms require more than large infusions of public and private dollars; beyond dollars, we need continuing analyses, discussions, and the desire of the interested parties to find the mean between desired reforms and the constraints of reality. This means that we must leave for tomorrow what cannot be accomplished today.

2

The Cascade of Dollars

Since the aim of this book is to document how new dollars were transformed into additional and improved health care services in New York City during the past two decades, we must set out the key figures that bound this period. But as those who work with figures know, even to outline the parameters of a problem often turns out to be difficult for a variety of reasons including the lack of data, the questionable nature of some of the available figures, and the need to take account of changes in the number and composition of the population.

To add to the complications, medical care in 1984 differs in many respects from medical care in 1964 not only in terms of what physicians are able to accomplish but also in terms of the resources that they deploy. The inflation that got under way in the mid–1960s and that has continued to today is a further source of distortion as is the fact that the Medical Care Index advanced considerably more rapidly than the Consumer Price Index.

These dicta should alert the reader that the figures presented below can only be reasonable approximations of the flows and uses of funds, but they are sufficiently reliable to provide a broad outline of the transformations that occurred in the health care sector over the two decades. Since the story we tell in this chapter deals with the gross changes that took place, the limitations of the data are not a major obstacle.

The pioneering endeavor to estimate the 1960 and 1970 flow of funds into health care in New York City and in fact the only serious effort to master the relevant figures, was undertaken by Nora Piore and her colleagues, Purlaine Lieberman and James Linnane, whose work was reported in 1977 in the *Milbank Memorial Fund Quarterly/ Health and Society*.[1] This chapter draws heavily on that report, as well as on a large body of unpublished data that Mrs. Piore generously made available to us for the present inquiry. We have also drawn on a recent updating and extension of the Piore analysis performed by our colleague, Dr. Matthew Drennan, under the sponsorship of The Commonwealth Fund.[2]

The most telling figures about the rapid inflow of new dollars into the system follow. Between 1961 and 1983, total combined public and private expenditures for health care increased from $1.8 billion to $16.2 billion or by ninefold. These figures are in current dollars and do not take account of the inflation that continued during all of this period. When the figures are deflated the increase shrinks considerably, from $1.8 billion in 1961 to $6.0 billion in 1983. On a per capita basis, the increase was even more impressive since the City lost about 10 percent of its population during these two decades.

Was there a striking shift in the characteristics of the population that might account for a sizable increase in the total use of health care services? The answer is no. Although the elderly, those 65 and older, increased by about 150,000 or by 3.2 percent, the number of children, those under the age of 18, declined by about 430,000 or by 3.8 percentage points. Hence a shift towards high users does not account for more than a very small part of the increase in real resources used.

Much can be said in favor of an analysis by decade if we seek to understand processes of transformation over time. A closer inspection of the period 1961–1983 reveals three distinct subperiods: 1961–1965, the years predating the establishment of Medicare and Medicaid; 1966–1975, the period of heavy inflows of new dollars; and the period since 1975 which was dominated first by the City's fiscal crisis and its aftermath and then by the increasingly stringent state controls over reimbursement.

Since we are concerned here with the transformational process whereby new dollars were converted into more and better health care services as well as into other outputs, we will focus attention on the 1966–1975 period. During the second half of the 1970s, the period of the City's crisis and its slow recovery, there actually was a decline of 2.2 percent in the quantity of resources used by the health care sector. In addition, in the five years preceding the introduction of Medicare and Medicaid (1961–1965), real resources grew at the rate of 3.9 percent per annum which was greater than the 3.3 percent average for the two decades between 1960 and 1980. But it is the 1966–1975 period that we want to inspect more closely, a decade during which expenditures in real terms increased by 5.6 percent per annum.

The substantial annual increase of almost 4 percent per annum in the years preceding the passage of Medicare and Medicaid reflected primarily the spread and improvement of health insurance. In 1961 total outlays for medical care amounted to $1.8 billion, of which private sector dollars accounted for 70 percent or $1.3 billion. In 1966 the share of the private sector was approximately the same, accounting for roughly seven of ten dollars of total expenditures for health care which had increased to $2.5 billion.

In the succeeding decade, 1966–1975, when the fastest growth occurred—in current (1983) dollars from $2.5 billion to $6.7 billion—it was the inflow of public sector dollars that accounted for most of the $4.2 billion increase. Of this sizable increase, the private sector contributed only about $900 million; all of the remainder, $3.3 billion, were public dollars.

The easiest way to summarize what transpired in the short span of a single decade is to state that the public sector, which in 1966 had accounted for slightly under 30 percent of the total outlays for health care, increased its share to just under 60 percent of the much enlarged total in 1975.

Further understanding of the relative contributions of the two sectors, private and public, can be achieved by considering the trends in terms of constant dollars and constant dollars per capita. In the critical decade of 1966–1975 real expenditures by the private sector increased from $1.9 billion in 1966 to only $2.0 billion in 1975, a compounded annual rate of less than one-half percent. In sharp contrast was the rise of public outlays which grew from $0.8 billion to $2.5 billion or more than threefold, amounting to an annual compounded rate of 12.4 percent, twenty-five times greater than private sector expenditures. After adjusting for the declining population, real expenditures from public sources per capita rose from $98 to $333, a compounded annual rate of 13.1 percent which implies a doubling every five and a half years!

This striking shift in the level and proportion of public outlays came during a period when the nation was enjoying a substantial increase in real per capita income, from $3,375 to $4,161, which amounted to a compounded rate of 2.1 percent per annum. For the first half of the decade, New York City's economy moved with the national economy, but in the early 1970s it lagged behind. Nonetheless, in New York City as in other urban areas, the enrollments and coverage in Blue Cross, Blue Shield, and major medical insurance continued to improve. And in addition to this improvement, the share of public sector outlays grew differentially.

These increases in public sector financing for health care must be placed against a background of New York City's large public expenditures for health care, a reflection of three factors: the long-term political orientation of the City (and the State) with its strong social welfare tradition; the relatively large numbers of poor and near-poor who lived in the City; the existence of the large municipal hospital system and other health care activities including many community-based health centers which were financed by the City. In 1966, New York City's public outlays were larger by half than the average for the rest of the country, 30 percent versus 20 percent of all health care expenditures; and a decade later the spread was still substantial. In 1975, public outlays accounted for 55 percent of all expenditures for personal health care in New York City while the national average had risen to 40 percent.

So far we have seen the magnitude of change in public financing of health care that followed the passage of Medicare and Medicaid in 1965. For additional background we must note that in New York State, unlike most states, the nonfederal share of Medicaid was divided equally between the State and the City; each was responsible for 25 percent of the outlays. In most states, counties contributed nothing and the entire nonfederal funding was provided by the state. In no other state was the county responsible for so large a portion as in New York. This particular intergovernmental arrangement in New York State (currently in the process of change) put unexpected pressure on the City's budget as its dollar outlays for Medicaid increased.

Table 2.1 provides an overview of expenditures in New York City by all levels of government for personal health care over the two decades, 1961–1980. Several trends are worthy of special note. Although the figures are presented in current dollars for the twenty-year period when the CPI increased about 275 percent, they point to about an elevenfold rise in total public outlays. The largest contributor to the increase was the federal government whose financing of personal health care in the City at the beginning of the period stood at less than $100 million while two decades later it was in excess of $3.4 billion.

Both the City and the State, each of which had spent considerably more than the federal government in 1961, had been reduced to minor partners by 1980 despite a five or sixfold increase in their annual outlays. Most of these increases had occurred by 1976. In the last four years of the 1970s, their respective rates of growth had slowed perceptibly.

Before we look more closely at the changes in expenditures by the principal components of health care, we should note that Medicare was directed primarily to broadening the access of the elderly (and after 1972 of the permanently disabled as well) to acute hospitals, and through Supplemental Medical Insurance (SMI) to physicians' services. Medicaid had a wider reach. Its aim was to assist the poor by paying not only for inpatient and ambulatory care but also for nursing home care, dental services, and drugs. In light of the respective thrust of these two dominant programs which served as the spearhead for the vast increases in public outlays for personal health care it is not surprising to find that most of the increased expenditures were di-

Table 2.1 Public Expenditures for Personal Health Care by All Levels of Government, New York City, Fiscal Years 1961, 1966, 1971, 1976, and 1980
(in millions of current dollars)

Source	1961		1966		1971		1976		1980	
	Amount	%	Amount	%	Amount	%	Amount	%	Amount	%
City	$235.5	44.5%	$349.9	45.1%	$685.2	27.6%	$1,160.1	25.4%	$1,366.6	21.9%
State	200.2	37.8	292.3	37.7	687.1	27.7	1,130.3	24.7	1,446.1	23.2
Federal	93.5	17.7	133.1	17.2	1,107.8	44.7	2,279.9	49.9	3,428.2	54.9
Total	$529.2	100.0%	$775.3	100.0%	$2,480.0	100.0%	$4,570.3	100.0%	$6,240.8	100.0%

Source: Data for 1961–1971 from Nora Piore, Purlaine Lieberman, and James Linnane, *Health Expenditures in New York City, A Decade of Change* (New York: Columbia University, Center for Community Health Systems, 1976). Estimates for 1976 and 1980 based on preliminary data from New York City Office of Management and Budget, New York State Office of Health Systems Management, and U.S. Department of Health and Human Services, Health Care Financing Administration.

rected to hospital and physician services as well as to nursing homes (Table 2.2). Between 1966 and 1976, total private and public outlays increased by about $6 billion; the private sector accounted for $2 billion and public outlays for almost $4 billion of the increase.

About half of the total increase of $6 billion was for hospital care, for which the public sector provided 80 percent of the increase. Another $1 billion increase went for additional payments to physicians. In this instance, the public sector accounted for slightly less than 40 percent of the additional payments. Hospitals and physicians' fees, it should be emphasized, accounted for about two-thirds of the total increase in outlays of $6 billion. There was also a sizable increase in nursing home care from under $100 million to over $700 million, mostly from public sector outlays. On the other hand, most of the increases for dental services and drugs which amounted respectively to over $300 million and $400 million reflected increased outlays by the private sector. The remaining large component, "other health services," which accounted for an increased outlay of about half a billion dollars, included such services as school health, federal non-hospital care, and in-plant industrial services and came overwhelmingly from public monies.

Another way of understanding the transformation that occurred during this critical ten-year period is to consider the changing contri-

Table 2.2　Public and Private Expenditures for Personal Health Care by Component of Care, New York City, 1966 and 1976
(in millions of current dollars)

Component	Total			Private			Public		
	1966	1976	Increase 1966–76	1966	1976	Increase 1966–76	1966	1976	Increase 1966–76
Hospitals	1,112	3,978	2,866	532	1,095	563	580	2,883	2,303
Nursing homes	95	714	619	38	134	96	57	580	523
Physicians	613	1,672	1,059	608	1,273	665	4	399	395
Dentists	188	496	308	186	458	272	2	38	36
Other professionals	71	145	74	70	99	29	1	47	46
Drugs	169	584	415	167	517	350	2	67	65
Eyeglasses, appliances	83	143	60	82	125	43	1	18	17
Other health services	124	604	480	54	65	11	69	539	470
Total	$2,455	$8,336	$5,881	$1,738	$3,766	$2,028	$717	$4,570	$3,853

Source: Nora Piore, Purlaine Lieberman, and James Linnane, "Public Expenditures and Private Control? Health Care Dilemmas in New York City," *Milbank Memorial Fund Quarterly/Health and Society,* Winter 1977.

butions of private and public dollars for each of the components. In 1966, outlays for hospital care were divided about equally between the two sectors, but ten years later the public-private split was more nearly three to one. In nursing home care, the share of the private sector decreased from two-fifths to one-fifth. If we add the two types of institutional care, the share of the private sector declined to 26 percent in 1976, down from about half in 1966.

The other striking shift occurred in payments to physicians. In 1966, public dollars accounted for only 1 percent of all physicians' earnings. It must be recalled that prior to the advent of Medicare and Medicaid, many physicians provided a considerable amount of free care to both ambulatory and inpatients primarily in hospitals and clinics but to a lesser degree also in their own offices. By 1976, about one out of every four dollars of physicians' earnings were covered by public dollars.

The situation with respect to dentists was quite different. Although Medicaid paid for dental services, Medicare did not. Hence, dentists in 1976 remained much more dependent on private dollars which continued to be the source of 92 percent of their total earnings.

Important shifts also occurred in the relative distribution of total dollar outlays among the major components (Table 2.3). The hospital sector increased its share from 45 to 48 percent of the total and nursing homes more than doubled their share from 4 to 9 percent, raising the total institutional share from 49 to 57 percent. Physicians' earnings dropped from 25 to 20 percent of the total and dentists' earnings from 8 to 6 percent.

Of the approximately $6 billion of new expenditures, about 80

Table 2.3   Percentage Distribution of Total, Public, and Private Expenditures for Personal Health Care by Component, New York City, 1966 and 1976

Component	Total		Private		Public	
	1966	1976	1966	1976	1966	1976
Hospitals	45%	48%	31%	29%	81%	63%
Nursing homes	4	9	2	4	8	13
Physicians	25	20	35	34	1	9
Dentists	8	6	11	12	0	1
Other professionals	3	2	4	3	0	1
Drugs	7	7	10	14	0	2
Eyeglasses, appliances	3	2	5	3	0	0
Other health services	5	7	3	2	10	12
Total	100%	100%	100%	100%	100%	100%

Source: Table 2.2.

**Table 2.4   Percentage Distribution of Increases in Total, Public, and
Private Expenditures for Personal Health Care by Component,
New York City, 1966–1976**

Component	1966–1976		
	Total increase	Private increase	Public increase
Hospitals	49%	28%	60%
Nursing homes	11	5	14
Physicians	18	33	10
Dentists	5	13	1
Other professionals	1	1	1
Drugs	7	17	2
Eyeglasses, appliances	1	2	0
Other health services	8	1	12
Total	100%	100%	100%

Source: Table 2.2.

percent was concentrated in three categories—hospitals, 49 percent;
nursing homes, 11 percent; and physicians, 18 percent (Table 2.4).
Seven percent of the total increase went for drugs and 5 percent for
dental services.

Striking differences can be observed in the distribution of increased
public and private dollar expenditures. More than three-fifths of the
increased expenditures of public dollars went to hospitals. The distribution of private dollars was much less concentrated. The largest
share went to physicians (33 percent) with hospitals next (28 percent).
Drugs and dental care together accounted for another 30 percent.

Since just under half of the approximately $6 billion increase went
for hospital care, a closer look at the changed patterns of hospital
funding should yield better understanding. Table 2.5 summarizes the
key data. The totals are not reconcilable with the figures in the earlier
tables because of the use of fiscal not calendar years.

As we have noted, in the base year (1966) private funds were still the
major source of funding for hospital care, accounting for close to
three-fifths of the total. A decade later private funds, although they
had doubled, accounted for only one-third of the total.

To shift attention to the public sector: in 1976, Medicare and Medicaid each expended close to $1 billion for the hospital care of their
beneficiaries. Their respective contributions to hospital revenues
were approximately 29 percent, with Medicaid slightly exceeding
Medicare. However, by 1983, Medicare had become the larger contributor responsible for 31.2 percent while Medicaid was responsible
for only 25.5 percent.

Although Blue Cross increased its expenditures by 270 percent

The Cascade of Dollars

Table 2.5 **Hospital Expenditures by Type of Hospital and Source of Funds, New York City, Fiscal Years 1966 and 1976**
(in millions of dollars)

Total Expenditures	1966		1976	
	Amount	Percent	Amount	Percent
All hospitals	$889.5	100.0%	$3,317.2	100.0%
Public	375.9	42.3	2,222.0	67.0
Medicaid			971.0	29.3
Medicare			956.2	28.8
Other			294.0	8.9
Private	513.6	57.7	1,095.2	33.0
Blue Cross	220.3	24.8	592.7	17.9
Other	293.3	32.9	502.9	15.2
Municipal hospitals	$312.4	100.0%	$1,042.0	100.0%
Public	291.7	93.4	889.4	85.4
Medicaid			471.0	45.2
Medicare			132.3	12.7
Other			286.1	27.5
Private	20.7	6.6	152.6	14.6
Blue Cross	15.1	4.8	49.9	4.8
Other	5.6	1.8	102.7	9.8
Voluntary hospitals	$511.8	100.0%	$2,108.7	100.0%
Public	84.2	16.5	1,240.3	58.8
Medicaid			482.2	22.9
Medicare			750.1	35.6
Other			8.0	0.4
Private	427.6	83.5	868.4	41.2
Blue Cross	160.1	31.3	503.2	23.9
Other	267.5	52.2	365.2	17.3
Proprietary hospitals	$65.3	100.0%	$166.5	100.0%
Public			92.4	55.5
Medicaid			18.6	11.2
Medicare			73.8	44.3
Other	65.3	100.0	74.1	44.6
Private	45.0	68.9	39.6	23.9
Blue Cross	20.3	31.1	34.5	20.7
Other				

Source: Nora Piore, Purlaine Lieberman, and James Linnane, "Public Expenditures and Private Control? Health Care Dilemmas in New York City," *Milbank Memorial Fund Quarterly/Health and Society,* Winter 1977.

over the decade, its share of total hospital revenues dropped from one-fourth to under 18 percent, and all other private payments dropped from one-third to less than one-sixth, which reinforces the earlier evidence of the rising importance of public dollars in paying for hospital care.

Proprietary hospitals in New York City have not played a significant role in the provision of hospital care; in 1966 they accounted for 7 percent of total expenditures and 5 percent a decade later. The more important and interesting comparisons are between the voluntary and municipal hospitals in the scale and sources of their funding. In the base year, 1966, the total expenditure of voluntary hospitals was slightly above half a billion dollars and that of the municipal hospitals slightly above $300 million. A decade later voluntary hospitals spent $2.1 billion, about four times their 1966 level. Of this increase Medicaid accounted for almost half a billion and Medicare for three-quarters of $1 billion, together $1.2 billion or roughly three-fifths of the total income of the voluntary hospital sector.

The growth of the municipal system was approximately half that of the voluntary hospitals; its expenditures increased by about $700 million, of which Medicaid accounted for over $470 million and Medicare for over $130 million. Another way to distinguish the experience of the two systems is to note that each received almost equal increases in payments from Medicaid but that the voluntary hospitals had a sixfold greater increase from Medicare—$750 million versus $132 million for the municipal system.

In the period of these ten years, the proportion of private funding for voluntary hospitals decreased from 84 percent in 1966 to 40 percent in 1976. The United States had avoided adopting a system of national hospital insurance in 1965 but by legislating Medicare and Medicaid it moved a fair distance in that direction. Moreover, the federal government continued to make a major indirect contribution to the expansion of private hospital insurance through tax benefits.

The comparison set out in Table 2.6 detailing the annual outlays of Medicare and Medicaid for hospital care in New York City reveals some interesting parallels and differences between the two programs. While both experienced substantial rates of increase, the growth path for Medicare was more regular than for Medicaid. This is particularly true for the more recent period when the State of New York made special efforts to contain Medicaid outlays. In 1971 Medicaid accounted for 62 percent of the combined outlays of the two programs for hospital care while in 1980 its share had dropped to 49.6 percent.

Total expenditures for personal health care in New York City came to $10.7 billion in 1980; the best estimate for 1983 brings the figure to over $16.2 billion. According to the New York State Department of Social Services, the Medicaid program in 1982 accounted for $3.3 billion of expenditures or about 20 percent of all health care outlays in the City.

There are several points worth observing. In New York City Medicaid has been spending close to $1 billion on so-called "optional services" of which the three most important components are personal care, intermediate care facilities, and drugs and sickroom supplies.

Table 2.6   Medicare and Medicaid Outlays for Hospital Care, New York City, 1966–1978

Year	1967 = 100	(1 + 2) Total	(1) Medicare[1]	(2) Medicaid	Medicaid as % of Total
1966				$115,053,784	
1967	100	$634,955,086[2]	$248,745,769	271,155,533	61%
1968	94	594,467,402	244,825,622	349,641,780	59
1969	106	675,491,619	316,086,163	359,405,456	53
1970	100	635,371,952	313,262,962	322,108,990	51
1971	157	999,798,386	380,356,211	619,442,175	62
1972	163	1,034,921,702	402,893,987	632,027,715	61
1973	172	1,095,170,188	458,376,875	636,793,313	58
1974	186	1,180,544,370	540,525,263	640,019,107	54
1975	225	1,429,779,963	666,001,384	763,778,579	53
1976	286	1,818,462,720	799,525,985	1,018,936,735	56
1977	277	1,760,706,586	862,158,827	898,547,759	51
1978	268	1,700,036,737	884,671,872	815,364,865	48

Notes: [1] Medicare disbursements shown are for enrolled residents of New York City aged 65 years and over, and disabled. Excluded are expenditures for care rendered to nonresident enrollees by providers in New York City.
[2] Includes 1966 Medicaid outlays.
Source: Nora Piore, unpublished data.

Inpatient and outpatient hospital care together accounted in 1982 for $1.5 billion or just under half of all Medicaid expenditures. The other large outlay was devoted to skilled nursing home care which amounted to $745 million or 22.5 percent of Medicaid spending.

Data on Medicare outlays are available from another source. In 1982 Medicare expenditures in New York City totaled $1.9 billion. Of this amount, $1.3 billion went for Part A benefits and the remainder for Part B for the 875,000 Medicare eligibles in New York City. On a statewide basis in 1983, 93 percent of the Part A expenses or $3,365 per patient bill went to acute inpatient care; 75 percent or $86 per patient bill of the Part B expenses went to physicians' services with 13 percent going to hospital outpatient care and less than 2 percent for laboratory services.

Even at this early point in our inquiry it may prove useful to consider the impact of these large additional inflows of funds, primarily from the public sector on three interrelated issues: the incremental services that were provided; the beneficiaries of these services; and the untoward consequences of these larger funds.

The passage of Medicare and Medicaid aimed to accomplish two primary objectives: broader access of the elderly to acute hospitals and to physicians, and assured access of the poor to an array of basic health services. The political bargain that the federal government made with organized medicine to encourage these initiatives was to promise that it (and by implication the states that joined the Medicaid program) would not disturb the preexisting freedom of choice in physician–patient relationships. The more enthusiastic reformers believed that with the new programs providing back-up funding for the two groups that previously had difficulty in "buying" their way into the system, the goal of a single level of care for all would be within reach.

With the advantage of two decades of hindsight, the accomplishments that followed the enactment of the new programs can be set out as follows: the elderly, who had earlier depended heavily on the municipal hospitals when they required inpatient care, shifted when they became Medicare-eligible and thereafter obtained most of their care from voluntary hospitals and from physicians in private practice. A high proportion of the entire age group moved into the mainstream of medical care.

With regard to Medicaid the evidence is less clear, first, because of the changing rules governing eligibility, second, because of the flow of people into and out of the eligible category, and finally because of the reactions of the providers in the voluntary sector to changing rules governing reimbursement.

When Medicaid was first established in New York State a family of four with two wage earners would be included if its combined income was below $7,000; with one wage earner, a family with less than $6,000 qualified. In June 1982, using 1967 constant dollars, the eligibility cutoff point was slightly under $2,300; in current dollars, $6,300. In the early years, about 1.8 million of the City's population were Medicaid-eligible; more recently (1982) the number has been around 1.2 million. Unlike many other states, New York State's (1982) Medicaid program has always included a large number of optional services which have not really been curtailed since the start of the program. But the shrinkage in the number and proportion of the eligible population indicates that the initial broad objective of Medicaid was not accomplished. Many of the near-poor, the working poor, and the non-welfare poor are not covered under the present regulations and have not been since the earliest years of the program.

The shift of the Medicaid population into the mainstream has been considerably more modest than that of the Medicare beneficiaries. It is true that voluntary hospitals today treat a higher proportion of indigents than prior to the passage of Medicaid. But the Medicaid population continues to make heavy use of both the ambulatory and inpatient facilities of the municipal hospital system.

Medicaid patients have encountered difficulties in obtaining care from physicians in private practice. The difficulty reflects the marked reduction in the number of practitioners in the low-income areas of the City; the low fee schedules adopted by the State; and the ability of the more successful practitioners to fill their appointment books without having to accept Medicaid beneficiaries. It should be added, however, that Medicaid encouraged the establishment of private clinics in low-income areas staffed largely by physicians trained abroad, many of whom have a limited command of English, where they provide one version of "private" care based on high volume case loads. Patients who present complex diagnostic or treatment problems at these shared medical facilities are usually referred to the ambulatory care services of neighboring hospitals. One measure of the limited access of Medicaid patients to private practitioners can be judged by the relative expenditures of the Medicaid program for outpatient hospital and clinic care versus physician reimbursement. For 1982, the respective figures were $396 million versus $105 million or roughly four to one.

Although skilled nursing home care was one of the mandated Medicaid services, and under the 1972 amendments intermediate care facilities could also be reimbursed by Medicaid, it can be stated unequivocally that no one who participated in their design ever contemplated that these two programs would consume over $980 million in 1982, only a little less than all inpatient care for Medicaid patients which in that same year amounted to $1.1 billion.

This brings us to the changing circumstances of the working poor, those not eligible for Medicaid but hard pressed to pay their bills when they need expensive health care. A rough estimate suggests a subgroup of between 1.2 and 1.5 million individuals. Many have some modest hospital insurance coverage, and they can usually pay out of pocket for a limited number of routine drugs. But if they confront a major episode of illness that requires the attention of specialists and lengthy or intensive hospital care they cannot cover their bills. Prior to the post–World war II inflation of health care costs and especially prior to the acceleration that set in after 1965 many of these working poor were treated in voluntary hospitals; recently they have had to use public institutions.

With the advent of Medicare and Medicaid and the subsequent inflation of medical costs, the system became increasingly "monetarized" in that voluntary hospitals and physicians, both of whom had previously provided a considerable amount of free and below cost care, now sought payment for all patients via private insurance, government, or out of pocket. This shift away from unrequited services to full reimbursement had particularly adverse effects for the working poor.

While the Medicare and Medicaid programs were the principal

factors in the enlarged inflow of funds into health care, all three levels of government—federal, state, and city—were the sources of additional funding in the late 1960s and early 1970s for community health clinics; substance abuse centers; family planning units; improved preventive services, especially for women and children; subsidies to providers that treated large numbers of the poor; extended home care services for the feeble elderly to prevent their institutionalization; and still other initiatives both short-run and quasi-permanent.

At the same time, the private sector, primarily through collective bargaining agreements, was a major conduit for enlarged money flows into health care primarily for hospital and physicians' services through improved benefits, mostly via major medical insurance which after a modest deductible provided the individual with 80 percent reimbursement for large expenditures of up to a million dollars and some without any ceiling.

Consumers also provided additional funding, often paying part of the cost of rising insurance premiums or purchasing Medigap insurance to fill in the lacunae left by Medicare. Consumers also paid out of pocket for all or part of the charges for physicians' services, ambulatory health care, nursing home care, home care, drugs, or dental services.

The gains in the quantity and quality of services, as we have seen, were greatest for Medicare beneficiaries. Still, the elderly who were on expensive drug maintenance therapy were not reimbursed for these outlays and dental services were not covered. Most importantly, except under restrictive conditions, the elderly did not have access under Medicare to nursing home or home health care services. Currently, only 1 percent of total long-term care expenses are covered by Medicare. The only way the elderly could obtain access to these benefits was through a "spend-down" provision which required them to cash in most of their assets before they would be eligible for Medicaid.

At the time when Medicare was passed, the general expectation was that the elderly would no longer have to worry about their health care. They would have broad access to what they needed and they would no longer risk becoming insolvent. But things did not turn out that way. Over the years Medicare has covered a decreasing proportion (under 45 percent today) of the total health care outlays by and on behalf of the elderly and even after allowance is made for the spend-down arrangement, the figure for their covered expenses is under two-thirds. On a national basis, the elderly still finance about 37 percent of their total expenditures on their own.

By way of summary, the facts and figures that we have reviewed justify the title of this chapter: a veritable cascade of new funds flowed into health care in New York City between 1961 and 1983, in current dollars from under $1.8 billion to approximately $16.2 billion, or more than an eightfold increase. The cascade was even greater when we recall that during this period, the population of the City declined by about one million, or by approximately 12 percent.

Even after the inflationary element is removed the outlays for health care in New York City in 1983 are striking. Total health expenditures, we have noted, amounted to $16.2 billion, roughly $2,400 per person, or close to $10,000 for a family of four. When we juxtapose this to the comparable outlays in 1966 measured in the same dollars, we find an increase of 115 percent on a per capita basis. The principal sources for the additional funding were the three levels of government, with the federal contribution increasing from 5 percent of total outlays in the early 1960s to 31 percent in 1983.

In Chapters 3 to 7 we will trace the specific impacts of this increased dollar flow on the municipal and voluntary hospitals, public sector health care, physicians, and other health care workers. All of these providers benefited—some very substantially—from the cascade of dollars.

3

Hospital Facilities and Hospital Services

This chapter looks at the ways in which the enlarged inflows of health care dollars subsequent to the passage of Medicare and Medicaid brought about changes in the structure of health care institutions and in the services which they provided. While Medicare and Medicaid were the prime movers, note must be taken at the outset of a number of concomitant developments that impacted the transformations in structure and services.

Among the most important were the following: the continuing advances in medical knowledge and technology that were pushing the system to an ever higher level of sophisticated diagnosis and treatment, particularly the major teaching hospitals which aimed to stay in the forefront of medical progress; the demographic and economic changes in the City and the suburbs, in particular the out-migration of large numbers of middle-class families from the City and their replacement by low-income groups, mainly in the Bronx and Brooklyn, with consequences for the private practice of medicine and an increased demand on hospitals for ambulatory care; the changing fortunes of the City's economy, notably the straitened condition of municipal finances which led to near bankruptcy in 1975 and which affected all City functions including its large health care programs; the increasingly prominent role of the State of New York in controlling the reimbursement rates for Blue Cross and Medicaid and in pursuing additional policies that had a major impact on the well-being and survival of hospitals within the City; and finally, the continuing importance of medical education and medical research carried out at the seven major academic health centers in New York City and in their affiliated hospitals.

The early identification of these institutional developments should serve as a reminder that important as money was as a transforming agent it did not operate in a vacuum. Demographics, public policies, and professional goals and values continued to be potent influences in reshaping the health care system.

The analysis that follows focuses on changes in the institutional sector (hospitals and nursing homes) for reasons which can be quickly noted. The purpose of Medicare was to facilitate the access of the elderly to acute care hospitals, and a principal objective of Medicaid was to assure that those among the needy who required acute care or nursing home care would be able to obtain it. Secondly, the hospital was the preferred setting for concentrating and using advanced medical technology. Thirdly, with increasing specialization, the graduate years of medical education were centered in the teaching hospital. Finally, with the decline of general practitioners in the low-income areas of the City, hospital-based ambulatory services became the principal and often the only source of primary care in many neighborhoods. For these and other reasons, a consideration of how the new dollar inflows affected the hospital is key to understanding the subsequent transformations in the health care system.

The impact of large new funding on hospitals invites consideration of changes among voluntary, municipal, and proprietary hospitals as well as among hospitals of varying size. With respect to services we will look at the trends in admissions and discharges, in total patient days, in inpatient vs. ambulatory care, in medical-surgical vs. specialized services. A critical concern throughout will be the extent to which the new dollars were translated into more and improved services and to identify when possible who provided and who obtained them.

One more preliminary observation: the fifteen-year period from 1965 to 1980 really comprises two sub-periods—the first, extending to the mid–1970s, was characterized by an open-ended reimbursement system; after 1975, the State's tightening of the reimbursement system coincided with the growing difficulties in municipal finances with significant impact on the large municipal hospital system.

Several reports of the United Hospital Fund provide the clearest overview of the changes that occurred in the structure and services of hospitals in New York City between the mid–1960s and the early 1980s.

First, a decline occurred in both the number of general care hospitals and the number of beds, from 122 hospitals and 37,300 beds in 1969 to 79 hospitals and 32,010 beds in 1983. Since in percentage terms the shrinkage in the number of institutions was much greater than in the number of beds, it is clear that most hospital mergers or closures involved smaller institutions.

Between 1969 and 1975, eleven small hospitals closed their doors, but there was no loss in total bed capacity which in 1975 was slightly higher than it had been six years earlier. The major declines in both the number of institutions and in bed capacity occurred in the second half of the 1970s when twenty-two hospitals with about 4,000 beds ceased operating.

From one perspective the shrinkage in the number and bed capacity of the hospitals in New York City in a period when the total dollar inflows into the hospital arena increased substantially must be considered as a counter-intuitive development. But as we noted earlier, changes in financing, while critically important, had to share the stage with other developments which were forcing the hospital system to contract. The City was losing population and the number of nonresidents who sought routine care in hospitals within the City probably declined in response to the expansion in the number and quality of hospitals in the suburbs. Furthermore, increasingly tight reimbursement controls together with changing neighborhood population dynamics made it difficult for many small hospitals, voluntary and proprietary, to balance their books. The pressure on them became even more acute when they had to make large capital expenditures to meet the minimum standards of the State to keep their certification. Intensified efforts were launched after the 1972 reforms of the Social Security Act to improve hospital utilization by exerting internal and external pressures on hospitals to discharge patients who no longer required acute care. The fact that hospitals in New York City had a much higher average length of stay than hospitals in other parts of the country indicated that reductions in beds were possible. Finally, the fiscal crisis in 1975 and its aftermath put pressure on municipal government to reduce its current and prospective outlays or at least to slow the increase, which led the New York City Health and Hospitals Corporation to look to hospital closures and bed reductions as a revenue-saving device.

With the exception of Downstate Medical Center, a modest-size general care hospital in Brooklyn, owned and operated by the State for teaching purposes, most acute hospitals in New York City operate under voluntary auspices; a significant minority belongs to the municipal system and a small number are under private (proprietary) ownership. In 1969 the voluntary sector accounted for just under three-fifths of all hospitals in New York City and just over three-fifths of all general care beds. The sixteen municipal hospitals accounted for just under 25 percent of general care beds, and thirty-four proprietary hospitals for 12 percent of the beds. A decade later the numerical configuration of institutions and beds had been strikingly altered. Although the number of voluntary hospitals declined from seventy-one to fifty-six, their capacity increased slightly and they controlled over 71 percent of all acute beds, a significant gain over the decade. The closure of three municipal hospitals accounted for the loss of about 2,500 beds of the public sector's 1969 total of 9,000 beds. As a result, its share of acute beds shrank to below one-fifth of the total. And the closures among proprietary hospitals led to a loss of 2,000 beds and a shrinkage in its share from 12 to 8 percent.

The United Hospital Fund's study, *A Decade of Change in New York City Hospital Services*[1] provides a wealth of additional information including the differential changes that occurred among the different types of hospitals and their bed capacities in each of the five boroughs. Interesting variations emerge from a study of the trends by borough, such as the relatively small decline in the bed capacity of the Bronx compared to a noticeable reduction in Brooklyn, even though the relative loss of population was greater in the Bronx.

Ownership and size provide important information for analyzing and evaluating changes in the provision of hospital care. They offer clues to the organizational strength and resources at the disposal of management; to the extent that scale and scope may be related to efficient operations, and to physician and consumer satisfaction. But we will suspend, at this time, further consideration of the structural axis while we focus on the changes that occurred in the provision of hospital services.

In 1969 the 122 hospitals in New York City provided a total of just under 11.4 million days of inpatient care. By 1975, their combined output was 11.9 million, a modest increase but still an increase. However, in the remaining years of the 1970s the number of inpatient days declined to 10.4 million or by 11 percent within the short span of four years. The number of patient days in the voluntary sector actually increased from 7.4 to 7.6 million but both the municipal and proprietary sectors each underwent a decline of about 600,000 patient days. As a result, the voluntary sector's share of total patient days increased from just under 65 percent to 73 percent.

During the decade, which was characterized, it will be remembered, by a decline in both bed capacity and inpatient days, the average length of patient stay declined from 11.3 in 1969 to 9.6 in 1979, or by 15 percent. This suggests that in the absence of any other change, the system was "producing" excess beds through this one factor alone. However, when we recall that during the decade there was a decline in the resident population and in the number of nonresidents being treated in New York City hospitals of between 12 and 15 percent, the shrinkage of almost 5,000 general care beds out of a total of over 38,000 looks less impressive.

Critical for understanding how dollars were converted into services is the factor of hospital admissions/discharges, both in absolute numbers and in the rate per 1,000 population. The general care hospitals in New York City discharged just over 1 million patients in 1960 and just over 1.1 million in 1980, or a 10 percent gain. Per 1,000 population, the discharge rate increased from 129 to 156 over these two decades or by over 20 percent. In 1980, New York City was hospitalizing its population at a gross rate slightly below that of the nation as a whole and since the City had a significantly higher proportion of older persons than obtained country-wide, its admission rate could not be considered excessive. On the other hand, as pointed out earlier, the number of patient days per 1,000 population in the City is considerably higher than that for the rest of the country, 1,480 versus 1,207, which puts the New York City rate almost one-quarter above the national rate. Taken together, the data point up that inpatient services increased over the two decades in terms of hospital discharges by almost 20 percent and in terms of patient days by about 11 percent.

These increases together with a decline in hospital bed capacity explain the continued high level of hospital occupancy, which showed a slight rise over the decade of 1969–1979, from 83.6 to 85.7 percent. While the voluntary system's occupancy rate was in the high 80s—between 86 and 89 percent—that of the municipals remained in the mid-70s throughout the ten-year period. In the early 1980s, however, occupancy in the municipal hospitals spurted due to increased demand and declining bed totals. In 1982, the overall occupancy rate for the New York City Health and Hospital Corporation facilities was 86 percent. By 1983 it reached 87 percent, approximating the level of 88 percent that prevailed in the voluntary system.

A second measure of the output of the hospital sector requires an evaluation of its ambulatory care, outpatient and emergency care visits. The total number of clinic visits increased substantially from about 5.9 million in 1969 to slightly over 7.7 million a decade later, an increase of 30 percent. But the comparison of these two years obscures the fact that in 1975 the total stood at 8.9 million, more than 50 percent above the level of 1969. The decade following the introduction of Medicare and Medicaid saw the hospitals in New York City provide a much larger number of outpatient visits, unquestionably stimulated both by the new reimbursement procedures and by the decline and disappearance of private practitioners in many low-income areas.

If the beginning and the end years are compared, no significant shift is found in the contribution of the two principal systems—voluntary and municipal—in the provision of these clinic visits, but in 1975 the ratio had moved from approximately 50–50 to 43–57, with the municipal hospitals' providing the larger proportion.

There were striking differences in 1979, however, in the outpatient visits provided by borough: in the Bronx and Queens, the municipal system accounted for 75 and 63 percent respectively; in Manhattan, the voluntary hospitals accounted for just under two-thirds of the total; Brooklyn was close to 50–50.

The other facet of ambulatory care, emergency room visits, increased modestly over the period, from 2.9 million to 3.3 million or by roughly 14 percent. The high during the ten-year cycle was 1973 when the total number of visits reached 3.4 million or some 17 percent above the base year of 1969. At the end of the decade, the voluntary sector had increased its share from slightly under half to slightly over half; the municipal hospitals provided 42 percent of all emergency visits, down from 49 percent in 1969 and despite the closure of many proprietary hospitals, their share had increased from under 2 to 4 percent.

If we add outpatient and emergency room visits over the period, hospitals in New York City increased their provision of ambulatory services from about 8.8 million visits in 1969 to slightly over 11 million or by about 25 percent.

Since our primary aim is to relate the inflow of new dollars following the introduction of Medicare and Medicaid to the production of hospital services in New York City, it is better to compare the early 1960s which predate the introduction of the new legislation with the early 1980s. Table 3.1 presents the key data for such an overview including a note of the year in which the number of ambulatory care visits peaked.

The dominant finding is that the inflow of new dollars into the health care system did not precipitate a dramatic increase in the number of patients treated. From 1960 to 1980 discharges rose by some 10 percent and the increase continues. The trend in patient days and ambulatory care visits, however, has been volatile. Up to the mid–1970s, before constraints were placed on dollar inflows, total patient days increased by almost 10 percent and ambulatory visits by 35 percent, but by the end of the decade both had been considerably reduced. Service volume trends in the first years of the 1980s have been inconsistent, with patient days rising and ambulatory visits declining.

This is an important finding but it does not reflect all that transpired. The data which have been reviewed relate only to the "quantity" of the output but an equally important consideration relates to changes in the "quality" of the services. Quality is always difficult to define and even more difficult to measure, but we must consider it in judging the effectiveness of resources used by hospitals or other health care providers.

A first clue to quality has already been suggested by the finding that

Table 3.1   Hospital Services, New York City, 1960, 1970, 1980, and 1983

Hospital service	1960		1970		1980	1983
Discharges	1.005		1.084		1.105	1.192
Patient days	10.481		11.518		10.468	11.690
Ambulatory care	9.062	(1965)	12.237	(1975)	10.848	9.923

Source: Figures are based on United Hospital Fund, *Health and Hospital Care in New York City, 1983*, and *1984*, and *Health Expenditures in New York City, 1983* (New York: The United Hospital Fund).

the hospitals in New York City were able to treat in 1980 about 10 percent more inpatients than wre treated in 1960 without a corresponding increase in the total number of patient days. And the subsequent rise in total patient days has been outpaced by the continuing growth in patient volume. This was accomplished by the more rapid treatment and discharge of hospitalized patients.

Reducing the length of time that patients remain in the hospital is, if other things are equal, an indicator of quality of health care. But other things have not been equal. We know from other evidence that hospital care in the early 1980s has a.much wider reach than it had twenty years earlier. It can do more and better for all patients, and for many it can now provide amelioration and cure where earlier it would have been unable to respond.

The third and most elusive consideration is found in the quality of life measures rather than hospital services—whether patients currently discharged have a longer and better quality of life than those discharged in earlier decades. There is a growing body of evidence that points to improved outcomes even though other factors, in addition to hospital care, also played a role.

Since there is no definitive body of data that reflects the changes in hospital use of resources after the passage of Medicare and Medicaid, the story will have to be reconstructed from diverse sources and, on occasion, inferences will be used to tie the discrete facts together.

To begin with, general care hospitals are customarily divided into the following principal services: medical-surgical, pediatrics, obstetrics and newborns, mental health, tuberculosis, physical medicine and rehabilitation, and skilled nursing. Since, as noted earlier, voluntary hospitals provided approximately 75 percent of all inpatient care in New York City in 1980, attention will center on them. During the post–Medicare/Medicaid years, the voluntary hospitals eliminated all of their tuberculosis beds because of the new drug therapy that could be administered on an ambulatory basis, reduced their obstetrical and pediatric beds because of the decline in the birth rate, virtually eliminated their skilled nursing beds, and kept fewer than 200 beds available for patients requiring rehabilitation because of the pressure on their acute care beds. The only major category of care in addition to general care which they continued to provide has been mental health. Twenty-one voluntary hospitals in 1980 with somewhat fewer than 1,400 psychiatric beds treated almost 24,000 patients with mental illness for a total of 450,000 days of care, which represented about 6 percent of the total number of patient days provided by the voluntary hospitals.

A simple illustration of subtle changes in the quality of care that hospitals provided during the 1970s is found by looking back of the stability in average hospital stay for maternity cases which was slightly above four days. By itself this stable average conceals the striking increase, from 9 to 19 percent, in the proportion of all births delivered by Caesarian section, a trend that was national, not solely local.

We noted earlier that most of the voluntary and proprietary hospitals that merged or closed after 1965 were small institutions; we can deduce that their disappearance did not adversely affect the range of specialized services available or the scale and scope of graduate medical education.

Another important development was the continuation of a long-term trend which finally resulted in the disappearance of most free-standing specialized hospitals. Of the twenty-one specialized service classifications in addition to "general medical and surgical" designated by the American Hospital Association, only five specialized hospitals survive in New York City—Hospital for Joint Diseases Orthopedic Institute, Hospital for Special Surgery, Manhattan Eye, Ear and Throat, New York Eye and Ear Infirmary, and Memorial Sloan-Kettering Cancer Center; their combined bed capacity amounts to 1,311 or 5 percent of all short-term beds. Moreover, all have affiliations with major medical centers.

One other important post–Medicare/Medicaid trend which affects the quality of medical care is the number and proportion of hospitals that are engaged in educational programs either as major training sites for one or more medical schools located in the City or with a looser affiliation with one or more of these academic health centers. Several other hospitals conduct freestanding approved residency training programs. At the beginning of 1981, most of the fifty-five voluntary hospitals and the fourteen municipal hospitals operated residency programs; thirty also provided clinical training for students of the seven medical schools located in the New York metropolitan area. An additional twelve hospitals have a limited affiliation with a medical school and five more are involved in graduate medical educational programs.

The structural changes that have been identified above—the closing of small hospitals, the substantial reduction of the number of free-standing specialized hospitals, and the large proportion of voluntary and municipal hospitals engaged in educational programs, undergraduate and graduate, must be considered a first indicator of an improvement in the quality of hospital services during the past two decades. A second and equally important indicator is the amount of personnel and other resources that a hospital has available to take care of its patients.

In the late 1970s Miriam Ostow of the Conservation of Human Resources staff with the cooperation of Blue Cross/Blue Shield of Greater New York undertook an analysis of a sample of twenty-four hospitals of varying sizes in New York City—voluntary (church-affiliated and other), proprietary, general care, and specialty care—to elicit the changes in their patterns of expenditures between 1966 and 1976. We will extract from this large inquiry a selected set of data that bear directly or indirectly on the changes in quality that occurred during this period.

A first point is that the hospitals in this sample increased their total expenditures by 305 percent during the decade. The medical care price index for the New York City–Northeast New Jersey area increased by 200 percent between 1967 and 1976 which suggests a substantial gain in real resources. It does not follow, of course, that if the hospitals added administrative staff or established employee benefits—both of which they had to do—that these expenditures would directly, or even indirectly, result in improved hospital care. But the opposite formulation is even more unlikely: that a 50 percent increase in real resources reflected in greater inputs of staff time, higher skills, more potent medications, more sophisticated diagnostic and therapeutic interventions, could have failed to produce a substantial change in the quality of care for the individual patient.

The analysis focused on seven major expense categories: household, nursing, special services (vide infra), general professional care (with subdivisions of salaries and benefits for interns and residents and supervisory physicians), administration (with a subdivision of employee health and welfare benefits), ambulatory care, and depreciation. The three categories that bear most directly on the quality of patient care are nursing, special services, and general professional care. These three accounted for 53 percent of total expenditures.

In considering changes over the decade, we find that expenditures for nursing lagged behind the average, increasing by only 261 percent, and special services increased at about the average rate or threefold. However, general professional care rose by 359 percent. Slightly more than half of the total outlays in this category went to salaries for interns and residents which increased by 386 percent; salaries for the senior physicians who supervised them increased by more than 1000 percent.

The principal functions subsumed under "special services" included operating and recovery rooms, anesthesia, delivery room, radiology, laboratory, physical and occupational therapy, EKG, EEG, speech pathology, cardiology, inhalation therapy, blood bank, I.V. therapy, cardiopulmonary lab, cystoscopy, renal dialysis, and nursing for these special services. During the decade under consideration, significant advances were made in all of these patient-care activities, some more, some less.

The hospitals in the sample were divided into five groups according to size with Group 1 the largest and Group 5 the smallest. A comparative analysis of the rates of change by major expense category was not particularly revealing although the following emerged. In each of the three critical inpatient care categories—nursing, special services, and general professional care—the rates of increase among the smallest hospitals, Group 5, were strikingly below those of the larger hospitals. The largest hospitals (Groups 1 and 2), on the other hand, experienced differentially large increases in their expenditures for general professional care on the order of 400 and 460 percent respectively.

The best evidence that hospital services were undergoing a qualitative change during the 1966–1976 period is found in the sizable increase in total personnel that occurred in our twenty-four hospital sample. It amounted to 37 percent, roughly from 27,000 to 36,000, at a time when the number of patients treated and the number of days of care increased at an average of around 10 percent.

While the nursing cadre showed the smallest percentage increase, 14 percent, over the decade, far below the average for all hospital personnel, it represented the single largest group of employees in 1976—11,400. When the 6,870 employed in special services and the 4,630 in general professional care are added to the nursing contingent the combined subtotal amounted to just under 23,000 or 62 percent of the total work force. The last two employee groups experienced gains of 66 percent or about 80 percent above the average increase for all personnel.

As foreshadowed in the earlier analysis, the small hospitals in Group 5 did not add many personnel in special services or general professional care. Only in the nursing category did they show a significant increase.

One surprising development over the decade was the fact that while all hospitals had had intern or resident staffs in 1966 this was no longer true in 1976 of any of the hospitals in Group 5 or of two of the four hospitals in Group 4. In contrast, Group 1 hospitals experienced a sizable increase in house staff of 87 percent. And the number of supervisors in the hospitals in the three largest groups increased at a rate of between 4 and 15 times the average gain in total personnel.

It would be wrong to claim more for this sample study. Despite data limitations, it underpins the conventional wisdom that during the decade large new funds flowed into the hospital system and contributed to the improvement of patient treatment and to an expansion of their educational mission. And these two major activities were mutually reinforcing: the pressure of a larger house staff with more supervisory physicians unquestionably stimulated the acquisition of more sophisticated equipment and the initiation of new treatment programs.

Other quality changes including long-term care can be extracted from a United Hospital Fund (UHF) report[2] which covered a total of seventy-six institutions, fifty-nine of them voluntary, sixteen proprietary, and one a state institution. Although the UHF had undertaken similar analyses in previous years, the earlier results are not comparable with the new findings because of changes in categories and other data incompatibilities. However, the 1980 results (based on 1978 data) can be used to highlight significant differences among hospitals according to the range of special services they provided and the scale and scope of their educational mission. For reimbursement purposes, Blue Cross groups the major hospitals according to the foregoing two criteria in an ascending scale from 1 to 8, with category 1 representing the largest teaching hospitals. The difference between the voluntary and proprietary sectors is reflected in the finding that the former had an average of 363 employees per 100 patients (inpatient and ambulatory) while the latter's average was 216. This means that the average voluntary hospital used 70 percent more personnel per patient than the average proprietary hospital.

A listing of the hospitals according to the Blue Cross classification disclosed that the most sophisticated institutions (Group 1) employed 431 persons per 100 patients while Group 8 hospitals had a ratio of 220 per 100 patients (see Table 3.2). Groups 4 and 5 had 331 and 303 per 100 patients respectively. The hospitals in Group 1 used 90 percent more personnel per patient than those in Group 8.

If we compare Groups 1 and 2 which provided a wide array of specialized services and educational programs with Groups 7 and 8 which had no interns or residents and a limited number of specialized services, we find the following contrasts in the percentage of full-time equivalent employees (FTE) by major functions:

The percentage distributions in Table 3.2 reveal striking differences between Groups 1 and 2 and Groups 7 and 8 with respect to three critical components of patient care: interns and residents and

---

Table 3.2   Hospital Full-time Equivalent Employees by Function, New York City

	Groups 1–2	Groups 7–8
Total personnel per 100 average adjusted daily census	431–390	240–220
	Percentage	
Household and property, administration and general	26.0–25.6	26.0–26.9
Interns, residents, supervisory physicians	9.4–12.0	0–0
House staff-nonapproved programs	0–0	3.2–2.7
Nursing	27.4–25.8	41.7–42.4
Nutrition	5.9–5.1	8.6–10.7
Special services	13.0–12.3	10.3–8.8

---

supervisory physicians, nursing, and special services. The small hospitals devote a considerably smaller percentage of their total work force to physician staffing and special services but a larger proportion to nursing. Since the percentage distributions tell only part of the story, it is necessary, in fact essential, to look at the actual numbers of personnel per 100 patients who are engaged in these critical care functions.

In Groups 1 and 2 there are between 41 and 46 physicians available to care for every 100 patients; in Groups 7 and 8 there are only 8 and 6 physicians, respectively in nonapproved residency programs (presumably mostly foreign medical graduates). In nursing, the differences narrow considerably: 118 and 100 nurses in the largest hospitals, 100 and 93 in the smallest. Since the patients in the smallest hospitals are likely to be less critically ill, the numbers of nurses suggest these hospitals provide as good if not better coverage than the largest. With respect to special services, Groups 1 and 2 employ 56 and 49 per 100 patients respectively compared to 25 and 19 for Groups 7 and 8.

If we add the three categories to obtain an overview of the numbers of professional personnel involved in critical care activities, we find that the largest hospitals have a combined total of 206 compared to 125 per 100 patients in the smallest hospitals.

The foregoing data are suggestive, not definitive. Hospitals which admit different types of patients need differing numbers of personnel to care properly for those whom they admit and treat. Furthermore, while a residency training program with supervisory physicians surely helps to increase the professional sophistication of the entire staff, it does not necessarily follow that all who are involved in the educational programs contribute directly and significantly to patient care. The point has been made repeatedly that much of the diagnostic workups in large teaching centers are of more value to those in training than to those being treated. But these caveats aside, there is a strong presumption that larger hospitals with more physicians and more staff provide a higher quality of care. We know that in the period following the passage of Medicare and Medicaid, many of the smaller hospitals in New York City merged or closed and the larger hospitals added more specialized services and more professional staff. The only reasonable conclusion is that the quality of hospital care improved, probably significantly.

Up to this point, the analysis has focused on changes in the volume and quality of services that hospitals provided for inpatients and ambulatory patients in the period preceding and following the passage of Medicare and Medicaid. But the full impact of how the additional dollars were transformed into additional health care services requires that we also look at long-term care. A small part of such care is provided by acute hospitals but the much larger proportion is centered in skilled nursing facilities (SNF) and health-related facilities (HRF).

In the early post–World War II era, Dr. John Pastore, then head of the New York Health and Hospital Planning Council, recommended that every general hospital make provision for long-term beds on the assumption that differential treatment settings under a single management would provide an optimal level of continuity of care for patients under efficient and economical conditions. Most general care hospitals did not follow the Council's advice; nevertheless, every acute hospital treats a broad spectrum of patients with varying needs, from those in intensive care to others who are convalescent, getting ready for discharge.

In 1965 there were sixteen long-term hospitals in New York City— twelve voluntary and four municipal with a total of 7,300 beds. In addition, there were about 765 long-term beds in general hospitals, and 225 long-term beds for mental patients. A decade later, in 1975, six of the voluntary long-term care hospitals had closed or merged and two of the municipal hospitals had shut down. The capacity in these long-term hospitals dropped to 3,000.

A special word about the radical changes that occurred during this crucial decade in the treatment of patients with mental illness. The number of hospitals treating mental patients increased from six to eleven but total capacity shrank from about 15,000 to 6,000 or by about 60 percent. This reduction was engendered by the new therapeutic approach that sought to treat mental patients in smaller institutions and to discharge them as quickly as possible to their communities. Coincident with the above was the increasing proportion of mental beds in acute hospitals; in 1965 acute hospitals accounted for only 17 percent of total capacity for psychiatric patients; by 1975, their share had doubled to 35 percent.

Even in 1965 most long-term care beds (other than for mental patients) were located outside of hospitals—in nursing homes, convalescent facilities, and the infirmaries of old age homes. About 3,300 beds were in the voluntary sector and over 9,000 under proprietary auspices for a total of 12,300 beds. A decade later, the total stood at 36,500 with over 25,300 beds in nursing homes and about 11,200 in health-related facilities. One in every three nursing homes beds was under voluntary sponsorship, but the voluntary sector accounted for 45 percent of the total of skilled nursing beds. Over the decade the voluntary sector expanded its total of all types of long-term care beds (outside of hospitals) from 3,300 to 13,300, and the proprietary sector from 9,000 to 22,500.

When we add all long-term beds in general care hospitals in 1982 (over 1,800) to the 39,500 in nursing homes, the total of over 41,000 long-term beds exceeds the number of general care medical-surgical, obstetrical, and pediatric beds.

Since one of the aims of Medicaid was to provide nursing home care for the indigent, the above data underscore that a sizable expansion occurred in such facilities following the passage of the new legislation. In 1976 there were 217 long-term care facilities in New York City of which 143 were classified as skilled nursing facilities, 69 as health-related facilities, and 5 were nursing home units located in general care hospitals. In 1977 the general care hospitals in New York City provided a total of 10.8 million days of patient care. In that same year the long-term care facilities provided over 13.4 million days of care, about 25 percent more than was provided by all acute hospitals. By 1982 the reimbursement pressures prompted many HRFs to convert all or most of their beds to SNF status, so that of 158 long-term care facilities, there remained only 14 exclusively health-related facilities for which a less advantageous rate was stipulated.

As we might expect, the length of stay of patients in long-care facilities was counted not in terms of days but in weeks, months, or years. For patients admitted to a skilled nursing facility, average length of stay totaled about seventy weeks. Patients admitted to a health-related facility in Manhattan had a stay just a little short of three years; the average for the entire City's nursing home population was about one and three-quarter years.

Medicaid paid for most care in nursing homes, accounting for about 90 percent of all patient days, and even in hospital-based long-term beds, Medicaid covered more than 57 percent of the cost.

Before concluding this analysis of the multiple changes that occurred in institutional care, that is, in hospital and nursing homes following the passage of Medicare and Medicaid, it is desirable to look briefly at how the new dollar flows were reflected in the total expenditures for hospital personnel, not only for the professional groups reviewed earlier.

The twenty-four hospital sample studied by the Conservation Project focused on the changes in personnel and expenditures between 1966 and 1975 and the results disclosed that expenditures classified as "administration and general" increased in dollar terms by 460 percent or more than half again as much as all expenditures. In terms of personnel, this category expanded more rapidly than the total work force; it increased by 46 percent versus an average of 37 percent.

But this does not tell the whole story. One of the striking developments which resulted from the availability of new dollars was the steep rise in the health and welfare benefits for the entire staff, professional and nonprofessional, which increased by 835 percent in the ten years and which accounted for $112 million of a $694 million total in 1976. In the latter year, three items—outlays for administrative personnel of $98 million, the $112 million of employee benefits, and the costs of household functions—plant, laundry, housekeeping and maintenance which came to $153 million—together amounted to $363 million or more than half (52 percent) of the total expenditures of these twenty-four hospitals.

We are now in a position to identify the principal effects of the enlarged inflow of dollars into the hospital system, including nursing homes, during the strategic decade after the passage of Medicare and Medicaid. We have identified the following activities that required and absorbed these additional resources:

- The general care hospitals admitted a larger number of patients, about 10 percent.
- These hospitals increased their days of patient care by over 10 percent, but in 1980 the number was back to the 1960 volume— 10.5 million days of care.
- These hospitals provided a substantially increased (one-third) amount of ambulatory care between 1965 and 1975 and although it declined thereafter, it was 20 percent higher in 1980 than in 1965.
- All of the available indices—size of hospital, professional staffing, range of specialized services—point to a rise in the quality of care provided by the hospitals.

- There was a sizable increase in the number of patients treated in long-term care facilities, mostly outside of hospital settings. In 1977, with 43,000 long-term beds, the system was one and a half times larger than a decade earlier. The quality of care was probably several notches better (though by no means generally desirable) as a result of the new sources of reimbursement (Medicaid) as well as the improved standards following the nursing home scandals that had erupted earlier.
- In order to provide more and better care, the hospitals (and the nursing homes) substantially increased their work forces, raised the wage levels of their employees, and improved their health and welfare benefits.

While the data and the analysis still leave many questions open and some unanswered and unanswerable, the major transformations which resulted from the new dollars flowing into hospitals and nursing homes have been traced. The additional dollars led to more and better hospital and nursing home services for more patients.

4

The Evolution of
Two Medical Centers

The thrust of the preceding chapter was the gross transformation in the services provided by acute hospitals after the accelerated inflow of new dollars that accompanied the establishment of Medicare and Medicaid. It will be recalled that reimbursement from these two programs came to account for between one-half and two-thirds of the total income of most voluntary hospitals. These sources of reimbursement also affected the flow of funds available for the financing of emergency room and outpatient care at voluntary hospitals but to a lesser extent than for inpatient treatment because of two factors: the considerable number of poor patients seeking ambulatory care who were ineligible for Medicare or Medicaid, and the relatively early imposition of a ceiling on the fees that the State of New York would authorize for the reimbursement of Medicaid patients.

In this chapter our focus shifts to a more intensive assessment of the ways in which two old, established hospitals, one in lower Manhattan, St. Vincent's, and the other in the Northwest Bronx, Montefiore, redefined their goals and objectives during this era of expanding medical financing.

While the larger flow of dollars into the hospital arena was the most striking change in their respective environments, it was by no means the only one. Some of the other forces which these hospitals recognized and to which they responded were changes in the medical and related social needs of the principal groups in their service areas, changes in medical knowledge and technology, and changes in the role of government as the public sector grew more important in the financing of hospital care.

The increased money flows created opportunities and challenges. They did not foreshadow and they certainly did not assure a particular outcome. In both the 1960s and the 1970s a considerable number of hospitals found it difficult, if not impossible, to continue to operate and either merged with other institutions or closed. But St. Vincent's and Montefiore were transformed from community hospitals into important medical centers. This chapter looks more closely at the ideas, decision-making, and actions that constituted the dynamics for the transformation of each institution, from conception to execution, and at the parallels and differences between them.

St. Vincent's Hospital and Medical Center

St. Vincent's Hospital and Medical Center, founded in 1849, is the third oldest hospital in the City, among voluntary institutions second only to The New York Hospital. The Congregation of the Sisters of Charity has played the key role in its establishment, growth, and management from its founding to the present, although in recent decades its board of trustees has included outstanding Catholic laity not connected with the Order as well as Protestant and Jewish members. Moreover, the Sisters have come to rely increasingly on professional managers to assist them in their administrative functions. A member of the Congregation continues to serve as President of St. Vincent's Hospital and Medical Center, the present corporate name which dates from the mid–1960s.

In accordance with Catholic doctrine and especially with the teaching of the Sisters of Charity, St. Vincent's has always defined as its central mission the provision of medical care under conditions that are responsive to the religious and spiritual needs of its patients, with a special obligation to serve the poor, the elderly, and the isolated. It considers itself first and foremost a community hospital and even in its recent restructuring which has brought with it a heavy emphasis on advanced medical technology and graduate medical education it has not shifted its focus.

In the decade before the passage of Medicare and Medicaid, St. Vincent's had a physical plant and a professional structure that were far from optimal to meet the changes that were occurring both in its own community and in medical and hospital care. To note some of the important tension points that were becoming more pronounced each year: about one-half of all of St. Vincent's beds were ward accommodations. The growth of private insurance had put a premium on semi-private and private accommodations and with the passage of Medicare, the death knell was sounded for ward care. St. Vincent's faced a major challenge to modernize its inpatient facilities.

At the same time it was becoming increasingly clear, especially in New York City with its large number of medical schools and major teaching hospitals, that hospital care had entered a period of growth and sophistication which required hospitals wishing to be in the vanguard to appoint full-time physicians as heads of the major services and selected subspecialties, enlarge residency training programs, and add depth to supporting diagnostic and therapeutic services.

As a community hospital, caring for large numbers of indigent and part-paying patients, St. Vincent's had relied on a voluntary medical staff to provide services without charge both to inpatients and to ambulatory patients. It was inevitable that tensions would arise when the hospital moved to expand the number of salaried physicians; this move was heralded by the recruitment in 1958 of Dr. William J. Grace from The New York Hospital to head the surgical service.

The growth of full-time or geographic full-time staff made possible the elaboration of residency training programs which in turn provided additional professional personnel to help care for both hospitalized and ambulatory patients. These new physicians replaced many of the volunteer staff who left when their prestige and control were eroded.

Another building block in the restructuring of the hospital into a medical center was the erection in the early 1960s of the Cronin Building for research with substantial financial assistance from the National Institutes of Health. While St. Vincent's never aspired to become a major biomedical research center, it early realized the importance of developing a clinical capability in selected areas.

Another challenge that St. Vincent's recognized and responded to during the past quarter century was the change in progress on the West Side south of Times Square which was its catchment area. In both its immediate neighborhood, Greenwich Village, and to the north and south, new apartment houses were being built and many brownstones were being bought and rehabilitated by persons with middle or high incomes. The population mix was changing in ways favorable to the continued financial viability of the hospital in that the relative proportions of poor and affluent shifted toward the latter. St. Vincent's recognized this shift and in erecting a new clinic building for ambulatory services provided for a large hospital-based private practice catering to full-paying patients.

In 1983 St. Vincent's completed the first half of its $145 million master plan for modernization by opening the Coleman Tower to provide up-to-date facilities for intensive and intermediate-level surgical and medical care. St. Vincent's had never been able to accumulate a sizable endowment and therefore had to undertake a special campaign to raise the capital which was necessary to obtain FHA financing for its modernization program. A considerable part of the money which it raised came from philanthropic institutions closely

Table 4.1   St. Vincent's Hospital, Major Divisions, 1966

Division	Bed Complement	Patient Days	Discharges	Average Length of Stay
Medical-Surgical	598	207,200	17,610	11.8
Maternity	62	13,800	2,760	5.0
Psychiatry	90	31,500	645	48.2
Pediatrics	78	23,500	1,540	15.3
Total	828	276,000	22,555	

aligned with the Catholic Church but the hospital has been able to attract some considerable sums from individuals, including many non–Catholics.

One of the striking aspects of the evolution of St. Vincent's Hospital into a prominent medical center has been its continuing focus on improved medical care for disadvantaged groups in and close to its vicinity. With the initial assistance of physicians assigned from the National Health Service Corps, St. Vincent's provides outreach and ambulatory care for the Men's Shelter at the Bowery and other centers for the homeless.

In 1969, in collaboration with the Visiting Nurse Service, it established an outreach and clinic treatment program in a number of single-room occupancy hotels in Greenwich Village and in mid- and lower-Manhattan, utilizing a three-person team composed of a physician, a nurse, and a social worker to provide services for many handicapped persons, including alcoholics, drug abusers, and former mental patients. For many years it has also provided ongoing medical backup for the Village Nursing Home, and was one of the first hospitals to assume such a responsibility for a facility outside its institutional framework. Recently it has pioneered a program to bring medical and social support services to many of the frail elderly (Chelsea Village Program) to enable them to continue to live in their own homes.

With this background of continuities and changes in mission and operations, we are in a better position to look more closely at the financial, utilization, and personnel data which together provide the details of the transformational process that occurred especially during the dynamic decade following the establishment of Medicare and Medicaid.

The profile of the hospital in 1966, the year when Medicare and Medicaid first became operational, showed four major divisions (Table 4.1). In addition, St. Vincent's was responsible for a large volume of ambulatory care. In 1966, it provided 140,000 patient visits, 67,000 of these representing clinic visits, and 48,000 visits to the

Table 4.2   St. Vincent's Hospital, Sources of Revenue, 1966
(in millions of dollars)

Source	Amount
Blue Cross	$5.15
Medicare	2.10
Medicaid	5.50
Other Patient Revenue	4.40
Nonpatient Revenue	0.80
Total	$17.95

emergency room. The remainder consisted of home health days, private ambulatory care, and visits to the Community Mental Health Clinic. Its net revenues in 1966 amounted to $17.9 million (Table 4.2).

To what extent was St. Vincent's altered between 1966 and 1980 in the volume and type of patient services it rendered? First, the hospital's bed complement declined from 828 to 788 during the decade of the 1970s as a result of major reductions in maternity beds (from 62 to 24) and in pediatric beds (from 78 to 49). These were offset by modest increases in medical-surgical beds and in the psychiatric service. In addition to the demographic changes that have been noted, the revised bed complement also reflected changes in average length of stay, changes in medical and surgical practice, and decisions by the administration to invest in arenas where the hospital had identified comparative advantages.

Against the background of a net bed loss of 40, or just 5 percent, between 1966 and 1980, it is noteworthy that a far more sizable decline occurred in patient days, from 276,000 to 241,500 or more than 12 percent. The trend in patient volume in this period also shows a decline (Table 4.3).

St. Vincent's strengthened its psychiatric services substantially and the resulting rise in total inpatient admissions, which was paralleled by gains in the number of outpatients, offset a dramatic drop in average length of stay from 48 to 20 days. Other services also experienced reductions in their average length of stay, notably maternity from 5 to 4 days and pediatrics from 15.3 to 9.1 days.

Table 4.3   St. Vincent's Hospital, Discharges, 1966 and 1980

Division	1966	1980
Medical-Surgical	17,600	15,300
Maternity	2,760	1,540
Pediatrics	1,540	1,360
Psychiatry	645	1,650

Table 4.4   St. Vincent's Hospital, Revenue by Major Function, 1966 and 1980
(in millions of dollars)

Service	1966	1980
Inpatient	$16.4	$73.8
Outpatient clinics	.6	4.3
Emergency room	.1	1.3
Other	.8	6.3
Total	$17.9	$85.7

The hospital increased its volume of ambulatory services from a total of 140,000 visits in 1966 to almost 170,000 in 1980 or by more than one-fifth. The expanding sectors included the Community Mental Health Clinic which more than doubled its work load with large increases in private visits and modest increases in outpatient visits. Visits to the emergency room declined from around 48,000 to 44,000 and home health days declined from about 18,000 to 6,000.

During the decade and a half when the total volume of patient services provided by the hospital remained more or less stable, its net revenue increased almost fivefold, from $17.9 to $85.7 million. Table 4.4 points up the principal shifts in the production of revenue by major function.

Another way to look at what transpired on the revenue front is to analyze the distribution of the increases from 1966 to 1980 by source of payment. The starting point is that net revenue was $68 million greater in 1980 than in 1966 which represented an average *annual* increase over the period of 11.8 percent. Table 4.5 presents the absolute and percentage increases by each of the principal payers.

Table 4.5 in conjunction with Table 4.4 points to the dominant share that Medicare and Medicaid contributed to increased revenues; together they generated two-thirds of the total new dollars, with Medicare alone responsible for one-half. The table also points out the increasing dependence of the hospital on third-party payers and the relatively small share, less than 7 percent, that grants and nonpatient revenues comprised of the total increase.

To expand and improve service delivery, hospitals require additional revenues especially in an inflationary period such as that which followed the establishment of Medicare and Medicaid. But to obtain more revenues, it was necessary for hospitals to spend more since third parties, the dominant payers, reimbursed them, with a lag, for what they had spent earlier. Therefore the interactions among the three facets of hospital operations—service delivery, revenues, and expenditures—must be sorted out to appreciate the dynamics of the transformational process that occurred at St. Vincent's.

Table 4.5   St. Vincent's Hospital, Increases in Revenues, 1966–1980
(in millions of dollars)

Payer	Amount	Percentage Increase	Average Annual Percentage Increase
Blue Cross	$11.6	17.1%	8.8%
Medicare, Medicaid combined	46.3	68.1	15.0
Medicare	34.2	50.3	22.6
Medicaid	12.1	17.8	8.7
Other patient revenue	5.3	7.8	5.8
Grants, other nonpatient revenues	4.7	6.9	12.3
Total	$67.9		

During the 1966–1980 period, hospital cost inflation amounted to nearly 200 percent. That means that of the $68 million increase in net revenues to St. Vincent's, $53 million represented no increase in purchasing power for the hospital. However, about $15 million was at the disposal of the institution to provide some combination of more and different services to those whom it treated on an inpatient or outpatient basis. We know from Table 4.3 that the number of hospitalized patients declined in the post–Medicare/Medicaid period. Hence the major use to which the hospital directed its additional revenues must reflect expanded outpatient care, a more intensive level of inpatient care, and/or greater emphasis on education and research. And that is what the detailed figures that will be reviewed actually reveal. The only other variable (in addition to plant improvement) that might have consumed additional resources were administrative costs which we will also inspect.

To take the easiest factor first—the volume of outpatient care—which rose modestly from just under 140,000 visits in 1966 to slightly over 150,000 in 1976. While the hospital's sizable outpatient work load was maintained and even increased with presumably some corresponding increases in the intensity and quality of the services that were provided, the bulk of the new resources that became available to St. Vincent's during the decade were not invested primarily in the expansion and upgrading of ambulatory care. We must look to inpatient care to trace the use of the new dollars.

Hospital expenditures can be differentiated along the following lines: expenditures for personnel of all sorts (professional, administrative, and housekeeping), and expenditures for equipment and supplies to treat and care for patients. As Medicare and Medicaid began to pay for the inpatient and outpatient care of many of the poor and the elderly whom St. Vincent's had formerly treated without charge or at much reduced rates—it established a charge ($5) for an outpatient visit only in the mid–1950s—the hospital was able to increase its staff, particularly its professional staff which enabled it to become an increasingly tertiary care institution.

Professional personnel within a hospital can be differentiated as between physicians and nonphysicians. The key components of physician personnel are the clinical chiefs and their staff appointees, and the house staff composed of interns and residents; nonphysicians include the nursing staff and a variety of health professionals who provide special services.

In 1966, St. Vincent's had 37 salaried physicians and 151 interns and residents who cost the hospital $585,000 and $465,000 respectively or a total of almost $1.1 million. A decade later it had an increase of 20 percent in residents to 181 and a total of 101 salaried physicians, which entailed combined expenditures of about $8.2 million.

The nursing service (exclusive of the School of Nursing) grew from 687 to 794, including 68 who were assigned to intensive nursing, for an increase of 15 percent. The total dollar costs for nursing increased from about $4.1 to about $11.5 million.

The third area of staffing change, which reflects the intensity and quality of service, is subsumed under the category "Special Services" and includes operating rooms and anesthesiology, laboratories, EKG, radiology and related departments and services. This combined staff totaled 326 in 1966; a decade later it had increased to 409, an increase of one-quarter. In dollar terms, the personnel budget for special services grew from $2.5 million to $6.7 million and total expenditures for these functions increased from $3.1 million to $9.6 million.

In sum, St. Vincent's expanded its professional staff from 1,201 to 1,485 or by 24 percent and its total costs directly associated with these professional activities increased from $8.3 million to $28.7 million or by 3½ times within a single decade. Even after we correct the dollar increase for inflation, we find that St. Vincent's was investing considerably more real resources in its professional activities at the end than at the beginning of the decade.

Hospital trustees and administrators have complained bitterly about the heavy record keeping and related overhead activities that the expanded reimbursement system has forced on them. The growth of administrative and general expenditures at St. Vincent's over the decade supports this complaint: there was a gain of 131 persons in administration from 240 to 371, and a total increase in expenditures from $3.4 million to $14.8 million.

The hotel services, of which plant operation, housekeeping, and dietary services are most important, underwent the lowest rate of increase in dollar expenditures, from $3.7 million to $10.4 or about threefold, with an absolute decline in the number of employees from 524 to 489.

A few more pieces of data will be examined before we summarize how St. Vincent's, a community hospital performing essentially secondary care, became a medical center with a wide array of tertiary care services within a single decade, although the transformation had its roots in the 1950s and the momentum has continued into the 1980s. Costs per adjusted patient day (a measure encompassing inpatient care and ambulatory services) increased over the decade of 1966–1976 at an average annual rate of 13.4 percent, with an annual increase of 15.4 percent during the first half. When efforts are made to extract the inflationary cost increases from the above, we still find a calculated "real" increase of close to 3.9 percent for the decade as a whole, with an annual increase of 6.6 percent in the first five years after the passage of Medicare and Medicaid.

It was on the basis of these additional real resources that St. Vincent's was able to develop a series of surgical specialties—vascular, neurological, oncological—and to broaden its radiologic capabilities, to participate in the Southern Manhattan Dialysis Center, and to become the principal support of Catholic hospitals throughout the City with the establishment of a neonatal intensive care unit, a burn center, a trauma center, a cystic fibrosis regional center, and a major psychiatric division including a large unit in Westchester County.

In the process, St. Vincent's expanded the number of its residency programs to fifteen and, in collaboration with the New York University and Downstate Medical Centers and the Manhattan Eye, Ear and Throat Hospital, sponsored three additional training programs in neurosurgery, urology, and otolaryngology.

. Concomitant with the intensification of its tertiary care capability, the issue of entrance into the ranks of the major medical educational institutions inevitably arose. The availability of public support for the expansion of medical education and the development of two new private medical schools by the Jewish philanthropic community in New York, the Albert Einstein College of Medicine and the Mt. Sinai School of Medicine, were further stimuli for St. Vincent's to consider following the academic route.

On several occasions the Board explored the possibility of becoming the principal teaching affiliate of an existing medical school or the nucleus of a new school, undergraduate or graduate, but it never undertook such a commitment. After the Archdiocese of New York assumed control of New York Medical College in the mid–1970s, St. Vincent's became its principal voluntary affiliate in New York City. However, the Medical College moved most of its preclinical and clinical activities from Manhattan to Westchester County.

St. Vincent's remains faithful to its tradition of providing care to many of the needy on the lower west side of Manhattan but in the last decades it has enhanced the quality of the care it provides by upgrading its staff and facilities. It has done this by attracting more specialists to its full-time staff, providing them with scope to expand and intensify their educational and service programs, and by broadening the sources of external support.

Montefiore Hospital and Medical Center

In 1949, the first comprehensive study of the hospital system in New York State, performed at the request of Governor Dewey, was published.[1] Montefiore was then in an early stage of evolution from a specialized institution, committed since its founding in 1884 to the care of patients with chronic diseases, into a general hospital serving the growing population of the northern Bronx and southern Westchester. The following year, 1950, Dr. Martin Cherkasky was named to succeed Dr. E. M. Bluestone, the long-time director of the hospital (1928–1950), and moved vigorously to speed up the effort that had been envisioned and initiated by his predecessor—the transformation of Montefiore into a broad-based acute care institution. Cherkasky's major strategy for accomplishing this was to enlarge the complement of full-time salaried physicians employed by the hospital and increase the number of attendings. In particular, he moved to recruit to the attending staff younger practitioners and especially alumni of Montefiore's graduate training programs who would admit their private patients to the hospital. Hitherto a relatively small full-time clinical staff had been needed to care for the chronic patient load; the hospital roster also included a group of distinguished specialists who headed its renowned neurology, pathology, and research departments. Its attending staff likewise was composed of outstanding clinicians, but they functioned primarily as consultants or in an advisory capacity, and their principal interests were in research and public service. Few of their private patients were ever hospitalized at Montefiore except as they too were in need of chronic care; for diagnosis and treatment these physicians admitted to voluntary hospitals in Manhattan, primarily Mt. Sinai.

The goal of elaborating the acute services at Montefiore which had been initiated by Bluestone was pursued vigorously through the decade of the 1950s by Cherkasky. The staff, which in 1950 consisted of 11 full-time physicians and 310 consultant-attendings, expanded to 64 salaried physicians and 516 attendings by 1960. The younger generation of postwar trainees was committed to a model of medicine characterized by advancing specialization, coupled with teaching and research, and as might be anticipated departments grew selectively based upon the professional talents, initiative, and organizational abilities of their respective chiefs. To continue to attract and maintain house and attending staffs of excellence, it was apparent to Montefiore—as to other older voluntary hospitals—that an active academic affiliation was needed. Since 1916 the hospital had had an affiliation with the neurology department of the College of Physicians and Surgeons (P&S) of Columbia, when P&S was one of only three medical schools in the country to sponsor such a department. But with the decline of chronic services at Montefiore, and more importantly the changing character of neurology, this affiliation was all but nonexistent by the 1950s. Under Cherkasky, Montefiore explored various possibilities for entering medical academia—establishing a new medical school on its own, or in collaboration with another hospital or a university.

By 1961, the year when a study was performed for the New York Federation of Jewish Philanthropies to assess the future of its ten member hospitals,[2] Montefiore was clearly the leading Jewish hospital in the Bronx and the logical candidate to become the principal affiliate of the Albert Einstein College of Medicine of Yeshiva University which had been established in 1955 and was located a few miles to the east. A formal affiliation agreement between the two was concluded in 1963 which provided for the appointment of Montefiore's full-time staff and many of its part-time members to the Einstein faculty. Both graduate and undergraduate teaching programs were to take place at Montefiore, including clinical clerkships for the medical students. However, both institutions retained their separate boards, and the primary teaching facility for the College continued to be the City-owned Bronx Municipal Hospital Center. In recognition of its new academic status, Montefiore was renamed the Montefiore Hospital and Medical Center in 1964. It was another six years, however, before a more integral affiliation was implemented. In the interim Einstein had built its own general hospital, The Hospital of the Albert Einstein College of Medicine, on the college campus. The Albert Einstein hospital had fewer than 400 beds and lacked the range and complexity of services needed for a maximal reimbursement rate that would guarantee financial viability. Although between them the two institutions controlled the majority of hospital beds and services in the Bronx, a number of factors militated against close integration. Differences in philosophy and mission (the more conservative, basic science/research orientation of the medical school versus the steadily expanding and experimental service orientation of Montefiore) and in particular the domineering personality of Cherkasky made the faculty of Einstein fearful of a loss of power and the erosion of traditional faculty autonomy in a more unified relationship. These overarching conflicts were played out department by department as well as at the institutional level.

The initial stresses and strains between Montefiore and Einstein were not resolved when Mt. Sinai decided to expand from a free-standing tertiary hospital into a medical school complex in the early 1960s. At that time the possibility of Montefiore's becoming a cosponsor or a major affiliate of the new medical school was explored, but this plan never advanced beyond an early stage of negotiation because of differences over location and potential staff dislocations. Logic and geography pointed to a Montefiore–Einstein affiliation.

The most potent force, however, was the reimbursement structure which argued for a single teaching hospital and eventually, in 1969, for Montefiore to operate both sites. When the original ten-year agreement came to an end in 1979, it was not immediately renewed. Once again the Einstein faculty wanted to go its own way and control its own teaching hospital, but once again administrative and reimbursement considerations forced the two to be reunited. In 1983, a fifty-year lease was negotiated for the operation of the Einstein College Hospital as a division of Montefiore Medical Center. Montefiore now has an inpatient capacity of 1,321 in its two divisions and controls 900 more beds through its affiliations with the North Central Bronx Hospital of the Health and Hospitals Corporation with which it is both physically and functionally linked and the Beth Abraham Hospital for long-term care.

Early in the administration of Martin Cherkasky, the decision had been made that Montefiore would move aggressively to become a strong general care hospital. The Trustees and the Director did not commit themselves to any one strategic plan to accomplish this objective but responded to opportunities that presented themselves. They kept their options open and when the negotiations with Einstein stalled or moved ahead at a snail's pace, the Montefiore leadership was busy exploring and taking action on other fronts.

During the postwar decades, the Bronx underwent precipitous demographic and economic changes, mostly for the worse in terms of economic viability and professional attractiveness. Large numbers of middle-class Jewish families moved to the suburbs and were replaced with lower income blacks and Puerto Ricans. Although Montefiore's immediate catchment area was the northern Bronx which remained relatively insulated for many years from the population exchange taking place to the south of it, it pursued a long-term policy of establishing itself as the principal source of high-quality ambulatory and inpatient care throughout the borough. This was consonant with the broader social view of the role and function of an urban voluntary hospital advocated and pursued by Cherkasky.

Montefiore aggressively pursued new federal and state program funds made available initially during the Great Society years for the purpose of increasing access to medical care services, and soon covered the Bronx with a network of institutional affiliations, neighborhood health centers, and other innovative health care delivery systems. Judged by traditional medical criteria, the quality of the services provided was undisputed. However, federal programmatic objectives extended beyond quality service delivery to emphasize "maximum feasible participation of the poor," the development of a degree of community political power, and opportunities for training and employment. In this climate Montefiore's virtually single-handed control of medical care in the Bronx was anathema to community activists seeking local control over service institutions. Conflict was frequent and resulted in a polarization which frustrated the goals of both. The construction of the North Central Bronx Hospital is a case in point.

Montefiore's skill in establishing and maintaining close relations with the public sector was one of the three foundations on which its long-term growth in size and complexity was predicated. Nowhere was this skill better demonstrated than in the collaborative effort worked out with the New York City Department of Hospitals to address the acute problems of the municipal hospitals whereby Montefiore contracted to take over the administration and professional staffing of Morrisania Hospital in 1961. This was the prototype of the affiliation system that within a decade tied each of the municipal hospitals to a voluntary teaching hospital or medical school.

When the New York City Department of Hospitals made plans to replace the obsolete Morrisania Hospital, located in the South Bronx, Montefiore donated land adjacent to its plant for the new facility to be constructed with the financial assistance of New York State. Cherkasky argued that only by having a physical linkage with Montefiore could the quality of the municipal hospital be assured. While there was considerable truth in this assertion, the abandonment of a major neighborhood employer in a declining area with few alternative resources made Montefiore appear insensitive to the health care and other needs of poor populations. The lack of public discussion of the plans for a new hospital further exacerbated political, religious, and ethnic tension. In the end, the North Central Bronx Hospital was constructed and now operates in close physical and functional integration with Montefiore as a major provider of services to the borough.

We have seen that collaboration with the City and the State was one avenue pursued by Montefiore to obtain much of the capital resources it needed to expand its operations. The skillful exploitation of the system of third-party reimbursement, which has dominated hospital financing since the passage of Medicare and Medicaid, proved a second source of strength. Cherkasky recruited talented administrative and financial managers who quickly became adroit in negotiating with the government, Blue Cross, and commercial insurance companies. Moreover, the administrative staff responsible for hospital admissions and discharges as well as those who oversaw the internal accounting system were guided by the fiscal experts in methods that would enable the hospital to maximize its revenues. Montefiore reached and maintained a high occupancy level long before any of the other major teaching hospitals. Finally, Cherkasky's long-term efforts to develop an academically strong professional staff enabled the hospital to attract large grants from the federal government and other sources to help finance the ever more costly tripod of research, training, and tertiary care.

In the long decades when Montefiore was primarily a hospital specializing in the treatment of patients with chronic diseases, much of its financing was underwritten by liberal gifts from its trustees and other benefactors as well as by annual grants from the Federation of Jewish Philanthropies. Such gifts and grants covered one-third of the hospital's operating expenditures in 1948; however, by the mid–1960s just before Medicare and Medicaid were established, philanthropic contributions accounted for only 7 percent of its much enlarged budget. The new revenues that Montefiore required to pursue its ambitious goals were not within the budgetary realities of the Federation, even with large contributions from its own wealthy trustees and other supporters. The proposal for affiliation and later merger of Bronx and Lebanon hospitals, both Federation institutions in the Bronx, with the Montefiore complex was not given high priority by the Montefiore leadership when it recognized that the long-term gains would be modest and might come at the cost of delaying the hospital's transformation into a major medical center. Rather, Montefiore saw many gains in a shorter period from pursuing aggressively its threefold strategy of close cooperation with local, state, and federal governments, skillful manipulation of the new reimbursement environment, and the steady recruitment of quality staff.

In the single decade of 1966–1976, Montefiore increased its total adjusted patient days, including both inpatient and ambulatory, from 318,000 to 521,000. This expansion of almost 70 percent in work load could be achieved only through simultaneous increases in revenues.

The hospital's total expenditures rose from $19.2 million in 1966 to $75.8 million in 1971, $135.1 million in 1976, and $253.5 million in 1982. The total cost per adjusted patient day climbed from $71.40 in 1966 to $259.50 a decade later. While much of these increases in expenditures, in total and per adjusted patient day, reflected the rapid cost inflation in the hospital arena, there is more to the story. For instance, during the decade, Montefiore increased the ratio of personnel per adjusted patient day from 7.23 to 9.95 or by almost 40 percent, a first indication of the greater intensity of services that it provided for its patients.

Nonwage costs per adjusted patient day—that is all inputs other than personnel—rose from $24.80 to $105.65, fourfold during this decade. Payroll as a percentage of total costs declined from 65.3 to 59.3 percent as a consequence of the greater volume of nonwage inputs.

On the basis of careful calculations made by a former associate, Paul Thompson, the index of the hospital's real resources use, corrected for the distortions of price inflation, rose by about half in the ten-year period. This was further evidence of the extent to which Montefiore was being transformed into a more sophisticated institution providing more sophisticated care to a more seriously ill group of patients.

Other data demonstrate concretely the magnitude of the transformation over the decade. The medical-surgical service, the backbone of a general hospital, increased its bed capacity from 483 to 1,044 or by 116 percent; this was primarily the result of the integration of the Einstein College Hospital. Turning to volume of services, in 1966 Montefiore provided 173,000 days of inpatient care for medical-surgical patients; in 1976 the figure had risen to 367,000. The most striking change occurred in the total number of inpatients treated: discharges rose 188 percent, from about 9,900 to 28,500. This greater "pass through" was made possible by a decline in the average length of stay from about 17½ days to just under 13 days. These figures clearly demonstrate the ongoing reduction of Montefiore's chronic care population.

Several other changes occurred in the number and types of patients treated. The gynecology department expanded rapidly and by 1971 provided over 18,000 days of patient care to 4,600 patients. In 1976, this department was reduced by about half as patients were shared with the newly opened obstetrical and gynecological service in North Central Bronx. The pediatrics service, opened in 1963, provided 12,400 patient days in 1966 and expanded to 38,500 in 1976; the number of discharges rose dramatically from slightly over 800 to some 5,700. In 1966 Montefiore still provided over 8,200 days of care to more than 1,100 patients suffering from tuberculosis; in 1976 the tuberculosis service was no longer operating. The other three divisions—psychiatry, physical medicine, and extended care—small in 1966, were still small in 1976. Psychiatry and physical medicine were each major departments at the Albert Einstein-Bronx Municipal Hospital Center complex; extended care was a small but very sophisticated program, concentrated in the Loeb Center, and was nationally recognized as a model for convalescent/rehabilitative care.

Montefiore had sizable physician training programs in place as early as 1966 when there were 131 interns and residents, and 61 supervisory physicians. A decade later, reflecting the advancing subspecialization, the staff numbered 273 interns and residents and 276 supervisory physicians and was responsible for an annual expenditure of over $14 million. [In 1982, the combined medical staffs of all divisions of the Montefiore Medical Center included over 700 salaried physicians (400 full-time, 300 part-time), almost 900 attendings, and a house staff of 622.] The routine nursing staff increased from 557 in 1966 to 1,222 in 1976, and the total cost of running the nursing services rose from $3.5 million to $18.4 million. In the latter year, 161 nurses were assigned to "intensive nursing" at a total additional cost of about $2.6 million.

As a result of the combined effects of a much larger patient load and a more intensive level of treatment, the special services required a steep increase in personnel, equipment, and dollar outlays.

As noted earlier, Montefiore's leadership early recognized the importance of strong administrative-fiscal direction and it is not surprising that the number of such personnel expanded in the decade under review from 338 to 567. Direct personnel expenditures increased from under $1.5 million to over $8.7 million. When health and welfare benefits and associated employee expenses are added, the totals spent for office personnel went from $3.4 million in 1966 to $31.0 a decade later.

It is illuminating to compare Montefiore's sources of revenue on the eve of Medicare and Medicaid with those in subsequent years. Table 4.6 presents Montefiore's revenues by source for the period since 1966. The most important finding is the dramatic increase in the share of government from 30 percent of Montefiore's total resources in 1966 to 66 percent in 1983.

The substantial improvement of physical plant and equipment that Montefiore underwent in the decade and a half after the passage of Medicare and Medicaid was predicated on two related strategies. First, through the erection of North Central Bronx immediately adjacent to its main buildings and under its professional supervision, Montefiore

Table 4.6   Montefiore Hospital, Sources of Revenue, 1966 and 1983
(in thousands of dollars)

Source	1966		1983	
	Amount	% of Inpatient Revenues	Amount	% of Inpatient Revenues
Total operating income	$17,520		$332,761	
Net inpatient revenues	15,585		267,287	
Blue Cross	6,544	42.0%	58,175	21.7%
Medicare[1]	2,388	15.3	135,866	50.8
Medicaid	—	—	41,293	15.4
New York City[2]	2,399	15.4	—	—
Self-pay, other	4,304	27.6	27,188	10.2
Philanthropy	960		1,864	

Notes: [1]Medicare began on July 1, 1966.
[2]New York City Charitable Institutions payments stopped with introduction of Medicaid in 1967.

obtained access to a greater number of treatment and teaching beds, and it was also able to rationalize certain services such as by adding obstetrics at North Central Bronx and expanding pediatrics at Montefiore.

Although as we noted earlier, its relations with the Einstein campus were never easy, in the long term, Montefiore was able to work out constructive subspecialization between the two sites to the mutual advantage of each, and there has been progressive integration of selected services. We cannot conclude, however, that Montefiore accomplished the complete metamorphosis it did simply by improved linkages with other institutions, particularly North Central Bronx and Einstein. These linkages permitted Montefiore to achieve certain gains in teaching and service but by themselves they would have been insufficient to enable Montefiore to become a major medical center. For that, Montefiore needed a substantial expansion and modernization of its own plant. In the two decades between 1960 and 1980, Montefiore improved its campus by a number of important capital improvements, at a cost of almost $75 million. However, its major construction program, first planned in the mid–1970s, will not be completed until the end of the 1980s having been delayed by the State-imposed inhibition of hospital capital programs in the intervening years.

In its formative period, Montefiore, like other voluntary institutions, depended on philanthropic gifts for capital expansion; such gifts continued in the post–World War II era but their relative importance declined steeply. The principal sources of building funds were twofold: grants and loans from government, primarily the federal government and the State, and the critically important provision in reimbursement policy which enabled hospitals to fund depreciation. This, in turn, enabled them to borrow from the capital markets. Montefiore made use of all of these sources, but none was more important than a strong assured cash flow which was the critical factor in convincing lenders of their creditworthiness.

A Tale of Two Centers

We have sketched the dynamics that characterized the transformation of St. Vincent's and Montefiore in the decade and a half after Medicare and Medicaid. It may be instructive at this time to take note of the parallels and differences in the ways in which each built on its own tradition and responded to the new environment.

From one vantage, the transformation of Montefiore in the post–World War II era was the more spectacular because it had first to shed its traditional mission of caring for patients with chronic diseases and become a hospital which provided general care before it could evolve into a major medical center and the principal teaching affiliate of a strong medical school. Both stages of the transformation were accomplished within approximately thirty years. In contrast, St. Vincent's was a general care institution at the end of World War II (as it had been historically) although it did serve a large number of patients with chronic disabilities, particularly alcoholism and mental illness.

Both institutions were community-oriented and sought opportunities to respond to new social needs and challenges. St. Vincent's had the advantage of its location in a neighborhood that was being upgraded while Montefiore was forced to grapple with economic deterioration and unprecedented demographic and social pressures.

St. Vincent's remained under the control of the Congregation of the Sisters of Charity although in time the Order shared responsibility with the Archdiocese of New York and a more broadly constituted board of trustees, the full-time chiefs of services, and a professional management staff. In Montefiore, the realignment of the leadership structure followed a different path. The trustees played a declining role because they raised a declining share of the total dollars, and they were confident that the institution was being ably led by the director, Dr. Martin Cherkasky, who proved repeatedly that he could obtain large public funds to support the conversion of Montefiore into a first-class tertiary care center. Although some of the trustees were uneasy about the boldness of these plans and most of them had discomfiting moments, nothing is as convincing as success and time after time Dr. Cherkasy could point to his record as the best reason for supporting his newest plan.

Despite periodic efforts, neither institution ever worked out completely satisfactory arrangements for becoming a true university hospital, particularly St. Vincent's which had not built up a strong cadre of biomedical researchers. Montefiore had far more to offer its neighboring medical school professionally and financially, and its role as a teaching affiliate is rapidly increasing in scope and depth following the absorption of the Einstein College Hospital and the continuing integration of clinical services among the three units—Bronx Municipal, Einstein, and Montefiore.

The transformation of St. Vincent's from a community hospital into a tertiary care center was made possible in the first instance by the large inflow of new funds that became available mostly through Medicare and Medicaid, supplemented by other federal, state, and city dollars. The Congregation, with the advice and support of St. Vincent's expanded board, and with the counsel of its full-time senior medical staff, was willing and able to upgrade the hospital, but insisted that this new emphasis should not interfere with the hospital's long-term mission to bring humane health care services to many groups in the community who otherwise would suffer from neglect.

Montefiore forced its way into the forefront of the major medical centers in New York City without a firm affiliation with a major medical school. It had had long-term ties with Columbia University's College of Physicians and Surgeons in the field of neurology, but the relationship did not extend beyond the one department. Although the logic of a close tie between Montefiore and Einstein was overwhelming, logic does not always prevail in the arena of medical planning.

In addition to these uncertainties and difficulties, Montefiore had two other major handicaps. Philanthropic dollars, which had played a large part in its earlier history when it became established as a major treatment center for patients with chronic diseases, became less and less important in a period when hospital costs skyrocketed. Moreover, the competition for the Jewish philanthropic dollar became more acute as Einstein and Mt. Sinai repeatedly sought additional funds for their respective medical schools. And Montefiore had to tread carefully in an environment with more poor people, more minorities, and more newcomers who wanted a piece of the political and economic action.

Despite these formidable obstacles, Montefiore became a major tertiary institution with a broad research and teaching mission. Moreover, it retained its strong community orientation as it sought new and improved methods of delivering health care to disadvantaged groups from the poor living in the South Bronx (the Martin Luther King Jr.

Health Center, the Comprehensive Health Care Center, the Family Health Center) to the prisoners on Rikers Island and the youthful offenders at the Spofford Juvenile Detention Center for whom it assumed medical responsibility under contract with the City.

Its success reflected first its strong leadership which perceived the possibilities of taking full advantage of the new dollar flow via reimbursement and which had no fear of playing in the political arena. The willingness of its Board to sanction and support such leadership was essential. Entrepreneurship is commonly thought of as a dimension restricted to the private sector. The evolution of Montefiore, under the leadership of Martin Cherkasky, is an illustration of outstanding public entrepreneurship.

Now the aftermath
Developments post-
Cherkasky

5

Public Sector Health Care

As with so many facets of urban experience, the role of municipal government in the provision of health care in New York City differs from that in other metropolitan centers. While many large urban centers including Boston, Cincinnati, Chicago, St. Louis, Houston, Atlanta, and Los Angeles have financed and operated a large public hospital to provide essential health care for the poor, none has a system with dimensions comparable to New York.

Public sector health care in New York is unique in scale and scope. New York City has had a major municipal hospital system in place for many decades, consisting of a score of major teaching, community, and specialized hospitals. (Even today, 1985, the reduced system includes eleven general care and two chronic care hospitals.) In addition, it has had a renowned Department of Health which operated a large number of well-baby clinics (at peak about 100) and thirty-five district health centers that monitored and treated various infectious diseases. For many decades, the municipal government also reimbursed voluntary hospitals for treating impecunious patients. Although the reimbursement rate at which the City paid the voluntary hospitals was set below the full cost, often far below, the public dollars that the City made available helped to keep the voluntary hospital beds occupied and provided these hospitals with additional revenue and, in the case of tertiary institutions, valuable patients for teaching purposes.

Moreover, the City hospital system has contributed major indirect support to several nongovernmental medical schools, the most important of which are New York University Medical School (Bellevue), Einstein (Bronx Municipal Hospital Center), and New York Medical College (Metropolitan). It has also provided major support through Kings County for Downstate Medical School which is part of the State's higher educational system.

In 1961, the City took the first step in a purportedly modest program which by 1966 absorbed $84 million, or about one-third of the Hospital Department's total budget. It entered into affiliation contracts with large teaching hospitals and medical schools to obtain house staff and supervisory physicians whom its municipal hospitals could no longer attract on their own. Able graduates of U.S. medical schools had numerous choices in selecting hospitals in which to pursue residency training and, because of the accelerating trend towards specialization, they opted for institutions which offered strong specialty and subspecialty training programs. Most of the municipal hospitals had lost out in the competition for house staff and the then Commissioner of Hospitals, Dr. Ray Trussell, saw the affiliation contract as the answer to an otherwise insoluble dilemma. The major teaching hospitals that decided to cooperate with the City also saw advantages in these contracts. The new linkage made it possible to enlarge their graduate training programs: they had a new source of income which would enable them to add to their staffs of supervisory physicians; and in certain locations, they could direct the flow of admissions of many low-income patients to their affiliates.

At the end of World War II, municipal government broadened its concern for the health care of its citizenry through major support for the newly established Health Insurance Plan (HIP), a prepayment plan which was designed largely for City employees and their families.

An inclusive listing of the range of the health care services provided by local government prior to the passage of Medicare and Medicaid would have to note the leadership of the Department of Health in operating various preventive and therapeutic programs funded by the state and federal government, such as those directed toward crippled children, maternal and child health, and mental health. Local government had also made a limited but significant contribution to the long-term care of needy patients who were suffering from chronic illnesses and the disabilities of old age. While the number of beds never met the demand and the quality of care was often criticized, local government made some effort to respond to the needs of these vulnerable groups.

One unequivocal conclusion emerges from this attenuated review: the public sector in New York (primarily municipal government) had a record of greater concern for and responsiveness to the health needs of its population, particularly the needs of the large numbers of the City's poor, than any other metropolis.

There is another side to local government's involvement in the health care of the poor and the medically indigent which we will review in order to see the whole picture. Despite repeated studies and reports by commissioners, committees, and experts which highlighted the inequities and inefficiencies of the parallel operation of two major hospital systems, one voluntary and one municipal, the leadership in both sectors eschewed close coordination and would not contemplate outright merger.

The reasons that repeated studies did not lead to action can be readily appreciated. The trustees of the major voluntary hospitals took pride in their institutions' being at the cutting edge of modern medicine, providing a superior level of care to their patients. They had neither the desire nor the philanthropic resources to increase their potential liabilities by assuming an expanded role in providing hospital and ambulatory care for much larger numbers of the poor. They were unwilling to enter into any arrangements with local government which would broaden their commitments since they were skeptical of the stability of City policy, particularly after the election of a new mayor.

The municipal leadership was also constrained in moving toward a merged system. It realized that even the best endowed voluntary hospital could not assume large continuing commitments for the care of the poor without much larger municipal subsidies. Moreover, greater reliance on the voluntary sector might demand steeply increased municipal outlays since costs in voluntary hospitals tended to be higher, often much higher than in the municipal system. By continuing to be a provider of last resort, local politicians realized that they were in a better position to keep control over the size of their future commitments. Finally, the large numbers of jobs in municipal hospitals represented an asset that no politician was willing to sacrifice. They provided substantial employment for local constituents, and they were a rich source of patronage appointments.

The uneasy balance between the two systems, long characteristic of the City's history, was shored up by the affiliation contracts of the early 1960s. There was one prestigious commission (Piel, 1967) which again advocated closer coordination through regionalization. Nevertheless, after Medicare and Medicaid were passed, the two systems were set to continue on their own. It soon became clear, however, that the large infusion of new dollars which provided more scope for hospital initiatives and enlarged the options for patients in turn stimulated new forms of entrepreneurial activity among physicians and nursing home operators, created opportunities for trade unions to organize and bargain more effectively for health care workers, and would eventually undermine the preexistent environment.

Before looking more closely at the impact of the new dollar inflows on the structure and functioning of the public sector health care delivery system, we will call attention to a number of developments affecting the needs of the poor for whose care the system was primarily responsible.

Changes in the population profile indicated that the City lost about

800,000 persons, roughly 10 percent of its total residents, during the 1970s. This was the first decade in the City's history in which the census reported a significant decline. The City had been at or around the 8 million mark since the 1930s.

More directly relevant were the numbers and proportions of persons at or below the poverty level. Despite the shrinkage in the total population, the numbers living in poverty increased from 1.2 million to 1.4 million or by just under 15 percent. This is the population for whom local government provided medical care. Children accounted for 90,000 of the 227,000 additional poor persons, or 40 percent of the total increase in the poverty group. Despite widespread impressions to the contrary, the number of the needy elderly declined substantially over the decade from 206,000 to 130,000, or by 37 percent, reflecting primarily the marked improvements in Social Security benefits and especially their indexing for inflation.

These gross data on population changes and income fail to reveal two correlated developments: the changing racial-ethnic distribution had resulted in a steep rise in the black and Hispanic population; in 1984 they represented about 40 percent of the City's total population, up from 21.8 percent in 1960. Moreover, racial and ethnic minorities have become the dominant or sole population in neighborhoods which previously were white enclaves. The local hospitals in these neighborhoods have been under increasing pressure both because there are fewer paying patients and because leadership and financial support were withdrawn as the former population moved away.

A related aspect of neighborhood change has been the reduction and, in some instances, the almost complete disappearance of physicians in private practice who used to provide primary care for a modest fee to many of the area's residents. As they relocated, retired, or died, new physicians did not move in and the local population became increasingly dependent on their neighboring hospital, voluntary or municipal.

In the first flush of Medicaid funding, both the state and local government sought to enroll as many potentially eligible persons as possible with a target of approximately one-third of the population. People were encouraged to enroll and were given information about how and when to do so by radio, bulletins, and subway advertisements. The enrollment drive was still under way in 1968–1969 when the State Legislature decided to tighten the conditions governing eligibility.

New dollars flowing into the system from both Medicaid and Medicare stimulated the rise in health care costs. When the State stepped in to constrain Medicaid costs by reducing enrollments and tightening up on reimbursements, it left a large number of the "working poor" in a worse position than formerly. The voluntary hospitals which had monetarized their system to the extent of paying physicians for services they provided to the poor were no longer able to treat as many nonpaying and part-paying patients with the consequence that many of them had to seek care from public hospitals.

By the late 1960s and early 1970s, the State of New York had assumed a more active role in controlling reimbursement rates for Medicaid and Blue Cross patients, in setting standards for bed utilization, and in other ways slowing the rate of increase in hospital and health care expenditures. These several State actions put additional strains on the municipal health care budget. To make matters worse, Blue Cross pursued a policy of reimbursing municipal hospitals at an unfavorable rate and in many instances because of faulty billing systems, municipal hospitals were not reimbursed for the Blue Cross patients whom they treated.

In 1970, at the request of the mayor of New York City, the State Legislature passed a bill establishing the New York City Health and Hospitals Corporation (HHC). The aim of the new legislation was to provide greater managerial freedom for the new corporation to run the municipal hospitals without constant interference from the multiple municipal departments; at the same time the legislation would insure that through his appointment power (two-thirds of the board), the mayor would control the new corporation.

The new organization was just getting into its stride and fulfilling at least some small part of the expectations that accompanied its establishment when the City of New York came face to face with its devastating fiscal crisis in the spring of 1975. At that point, and for several years thereafter, the mayor and the Board of Estimate had no option but to concentrate on bringing the municipal budget into balance. Budget cutting was a major obligation. During the ensuing years of retrenchment, the large number of employees working in the municipal hospitals became a prime target.

We are now in a better position to look at both the enlarged dollar flows that followed the introduction of Medicare and Medicaid and the subsequent expenditures of the public sector for health care. The best way to obtain perspective on the dollar flows as they impacted public sector health care is to draw on Nora Piore's classic article in which she and her collaborators presented most of the critical figures. Piore reviewed what had transpired during the period from shortly before the passage of Medicare and Medicaid to 1975 when most of the impacts on the municipal health care system had taken place.

In fiscal year 1961, after collections from and on behalf of patients, the City had to raise from its own tax levy funds $218 million to cover unrequited outlays for all forms of personal health care. In fiscal year

1966, the total had risen by half to $326 million. In the next quinquennium, it had almost doubled to $641 million and by 1975 it stood at $1.2 billion representing over a fivefold increase over the base year of 1961.

Through the establishment of Medicare in 1966, the federal government assumed responsibility for a high proportion of all the health care expenses of the elderly, and with the amendments of 1972, also covered major health care costs for the blind and the disabled. The large increases in municipal expenditures for health care are therefore surprising, particularly in light of the new dollar flows from Medicaid. True, New York State had the unusual requirement that local government had to contribute 25 percent towards the costs of Medicaid but that still left the federal and the state governments as the source for three of every four Medicaid dollars.

In fiscal year 1966, the City spent on health care slightly over half a billion dollars ($524 million) from its own tax levy funds and federal and State intergovernmental transfers. Two-thirds of this amount went for hospital care, $266 million for its own system, and $81 million in subsidy for voluntary hospitals that cared for patients who were the City's responsibility. The Department of Welfare spent $53 million mostly on long-term care for the poor and the disabled. The remaining allocations were to: Community Mental Health Board, $48 million; employee benefits, $32 million; Department of Health, $23 million; and debt service, $21 million.

The foregoing provides an overview of the public dollar outlays that passed through the municipal budget but in addition considerable, if smaller, amounts were spent in New York City directly by State government—$176 million, primarily through the Department of Mental Hygiene for inpatient psychiatric treatment—and $66 million by the federal government of which about two-thirds represented expenditures of the Veterans Administration.

If we combine all "public dollars" spent by City, State, and federal government for personal health care in New York City in 1966, we find that of the total of $700 million, $580 million or about 83 percent was spent for hospital care. Nursing home care amounted to $40 million, less than 6 percent. Only $4.4 million went for physicians' services and $3.7 million for drugs and appliances, small proportions indeed.

During the era that followed the passage of Medicare, there was, in addition to direct budgetary allocations for health care services, a significant flow of federal funds that bypassed State and local government, namely, the reimbursement payments for inpatient and ambulatory care for Medicare beneficiaries. These funds must be added to the other governmental outlays to obtain a view of total public dollar expenditures for health care.

The most illuminating contrast is the distribution of all public health care dollars between fiscal year 1966 when they totaled $700 million and fiscal year 1975 when they stood at slightly above $4 billion. Hospital care continued to dominate the expenditures, but despite a large absolute increase of about $2 billion, the relative proportion allocated to hospitals declined from 83 to 63 percent. The most striking gain occurred in physicians' services. In the base year (1966) $4.4 million public dollars had recompensed physicians for their services; in 1975 the figure was $362 million which represented a multiple of more than 80! A less steep but still substantial increase occurred in the combined categories of drugs and appliances, which went from $3.7 million to $133 million or almost fortyfold.

The other important development reflected the increased outlays for nursing home care which rose from $40 million to $347 million, or more than eightfold. The catchall category of "other health services" increased from $69 million to $582 million, also more than eightfold.

Table 5.1, adopted from Piore, provides an overview of the distribution of the increased flow of public dollars over the critical decade.

The changed pattern of distribution can easily be summarized: of the more than $3.3 billion additional public dollars, almost $2 billion went to hospitals for inpatient and ambulatory care. Physicians and nursing homes each accounted for sizable increases, and the miscellaneous categories absorbed an additional two-thirds of $1 billion.

These large increases in dollar flows into the health care system, primarily through the two entitlement programs, Medicare and Medicaid, with their heavy but not exclusive focus on the financing of hospital care, was certain to change how, where, and from whom patients received care. The changes in the patterns of health care that followed upon the new financing are set out below:

- The number of hospital admissions for patients aged 65 or older increased substantially, from 222 per 1,000 in 1958 to 284 per 1,000 in 1980. Despite the extensive provisions that local government had had in place to provide hospital care for the needy prior to the new financing arrangements, the elderly were not being admitted to acute hospitals to the extent that their conditions warranted. The new financing schemes may have encouraged physicians to admit elderly patients with certain conditions who could have been treated on an ambulatory basis, but the sizable rise in the admissions rate for the elderly is

Table 5.1 Distribution of Public Dollars for Medical Care, New York City, 1966 and 1975
(in millions of dollars)

	1966	1975	Increase
Hospital care	$580	$2,538	$1,958
Physician services	4	362	358
Nursing home care	40	347	307
Drugs, appliances	4	133	129
Other health services	69	582	513
All other	3	45	42
Total	$700	$4,007	$3,307

presumptive evidence that the federal and State legislators were on the right track when they lowered the financial barriers.

• The new legislation aimed at increasing the degrees of freedom available to patients to choose physicians and other health care providers. The data demonstrate that this objective was met for patients requiring inpatient treatment. The proportion of the 65 or older who continued to be treated in municipal hospitals declined from 36.9 percent in 1958 to 13.5 percent in 1980.

• Even among the poor, as distinct from the elderly, there was a clear shift out of municipal into voluntary hospitals although a high proportion of all Medicaid patients continue to be treated in the municipal system.

• To complete the account of the impacts of Medicaid on the extent to which the poor obtained expanded access to hospital care, we find the following contrast between 1964 and 1980: the hospitalization rate for persons living in poverty increased from 195 per 1,000 for 1958 to 214 per 1,000 in 1980. This rate is somewhat misleading given different definitions of poverty between the two periods.

Reformulated, the large inflows of new public dollars had the following effects on voluntary and municipal hospitals and on the elderly and the poor who sought inpatient treatment. Both the elderly and the poor obtained easier access to hospital care; more of the care which they received was provided in voluntary hospitals, and despite the large inflow of public dollars, the municipal hospital system became constrained on all fronts—beds, admissions, and days of care. The only reasonable conclusion from these findings is that the elderly and the poor, when afforded an opportunity to select the setting in which to obtain care, particularly inpatient care, opted for the voluntary system.

In ambulatory care, the trend is somewhat less straightforward and the outcome somewhat more equivocal. First, the total number of ambulatory care visits provided by all hospitals increased by slightly more than 3 million visits between 1965 and 1975, or by one-third. In the following five years, the total number of visits to the outpatient and emergency rooms of hospitals declined substantially; at 10.9 million in 1981, they were about 1.4 million visits below the level for 1975. To some extent this was the result of redefinition of service terms.

The experience of the public and voluntary systems differed with respect to ambulatory care. Between 1965 and 1975 both systems increased their volume of care proportionately with the municipal system accounting for just under 54 percent in both years and the voluntary system at the 45 percent mark. But in the late 1970s while the voluntary system held its volume of services at about 5.5 million visits, its share of the total increased from 45 to over 51 percent because of the reduction by the municipal system of 1.5 million visits from about 6.6 to 5.1 million.

One explanation for the decline was the shrinkage in the total population. Another resulted from the closure of several municipal hospitals. A third was the growing resistance of voluntary hospitals to treat a large a number of patients for whom they could expect no reimbursement. We must also take into account the presence in New York City of a secondary system of institutional ambulatory care provided by freestanding clinics and hospital satellites.

In a study by Diane Rowland and Clifton R. Gaus prepared for The Commonwealth Fund, we find in an accounting of $123 million dollars of direct federal funding for health services in New York City for fiscal year 1980 that an estimated $26 million was made available to help support thirty-two community health centers (mostly in low-income areas of the City) which provided primary care to over 230,000 low-income persons. A high proportion of the other $97 million was also spent on providing primary care services to the poor and the near-poor including a range of preventive and therapeutic services to mothers and children, care for disabled children, hypertension control, and emergency medical care. Close to $40 million was spent for the control of alcohol and drug abuse and for mental health.

The United Hospital Fund has estimated that there may be as many as 3 million additional ambulatory visits to institutions other than voluntary or municipal hospitals which, as we have seen, provided just under 11 million ambulatory care visits in 1980.

The other source of medical care available to low-income persons was the newly formed large multi-physician practices which were established in response to the new sources of funding, primarily Medicaid. Most of the elderly were not poor and the Medicare program reimbursed physicians at reasonable rates, offering them the option of not accepting assignment which meant that their patients had to cover their bills in full.

The situation with respect to Medicaid was quite different. Early on, the State set a low fee for physicians who treated Medicaid patients in their offices. Moreover, when Medicaid was enacted, many physicians were already working as many hours each day as they desired. As a result they were not motivated to increase their patient rolls. Many also realized that their middle-class patients would resent having to share the waiting room with large numbers of poor people. In short, most physicians in private practice turned their backs on Medicaid.

However, some entrepreneurially inclined physicians, especially those who were graduates of foreign medical schools, including many recent immigrants, recognized the opportunities that Medicaid presented. Using storefronts and other available sites, Medicaid clinics started to spring up in various parts of the City, in some locations as partnerships, in others as physician-owned corporations, in which physicians were hired on an hourly or weekly basis. Many of these clinics offered a level of care which, in the unsophisticated view of the patients who used them, was preferable to the care they could obtain at a neighboring hospital or from one of the remaining practitioners in the area.

In the middle 1970s, evidence accumulated that some Medicaid providers, not only physicians, were engaging in questionable if not fraudulent practices and legal action was taken against some of the worst offenders who had been billing for services not rendered. The Department of Health had to close a number of clinics because of gross infractions of the sanitary and fire codes. An analysis of the billings disclosed that a very small percentage of all practicing physicians in the City were treating Medicaid patients: some 10 percent of all physicians accounted for around 70 percent of all Medicaid billings.

The only way that large Medicaid clinics could make a profit was to establish and maintain a high volume. When these clinics were confronted with a difficult diagnostic problem, they frequently referred the patient to the emergency room of a neighboring hospital. And they tended to do the same when it came to treating patients for whom the time/revenue ratio was unfavorable. On the other hand, they could not be too cavalier without running the risk of losing support among existing and potential patients.

In the absence of a definitive study with adequate controls, the most reasonable conclusion about the middle range of the large Medicaid clinics is that they were probably no worse than, and because of shorter waiting time probably somewhat superior to, the ambulatory care settings of the municipal and small community hospitals that continued to operate in the low-income areas of the City.

There is less ambiguity about the impact of the new public spending on nursing home care for the poor and near-poor. Initially limited to skilled nursing facilities, the amendments to the Medicaid legislation enacted in 1972 broadened access to nursing home care by including health-related beds. In the ensuing years, there was a substantial expansion in the number of nursing homes, far beyond what the designers of the legislation had contemplated.

In 1966 the public dollars flowing into nursing homes amounted to $40 million; by 1975, $347 million; and in 1981 the Medicaid share alone amounted to $88.7 million to which additional funds from Medicare were added. The bed capacity of nursing homes doubled during the decade of 1971–1981, from 20,000 to about 40,000. Since nursing homes in New York City have been operating consistently at high occupancy, the increase in beds reflected a corresponding increase in the days of care provided. While more than half of this bed capacity is in proprietary nursing homes, most of the revenue of these homes and of those under voluntary auspices is provided by Medicaid and to a small degree by Medicare funds. Paying patients account for about 30 percent.

Both the costs and the quality of care provided in nursing homes vary markedly. After the scandals that surfaced in the early 1970s, the authorities tightened their supervision and as a result the worst institutions were closed. But since the list of patients seeking admission outnumbers the beds available, the authorities have had to act with circumspection. Moreover, with severe cost constraints in place, the reimbursement rate for Medicaid patients does not provide much scope for improvement. Only well-managed institutions can provide an acceptable level of care at the approved rate and then only if they pursue a selective admissions policy which limits the number of persons who require continuing supervision and care.

Let us now briefly consider dental services and drugs and appliances. Prior to 1966, public outlays for dental services amounted to only $2 million. In 1976, the figure was over twenty times greater. Increased outlays for drugs and appliances rose from under $4 million to over $190 million, a 48-fold rise within a single decade. The almost $600 million public dollar outlays consisting of "other health services" that Nora Piore reported for 1976 included a miscellany of home health care, general and special clinic care, abortions, transportation of patients to and from medical providers.

On the basis of the foregoing review, we are now in a better position to reach some tentative conclusions about the impact of the large increases in public dollars, from about $700 million in 1966 to $6.2

billion in 1983. Since the medical care index advanced by 300 percent over this period and since there was an increase of more than three-fold in current expenditures, we will try to point to the types and amounts of additional health services which were provided, and to who produced and who received them; and then we will consider some of the financial and related consequences that followed these high expenditures.

The total number of general hospital patient days declined over the decade and a half between 1965 and 1980, but the number of patients treated increased and the intensity of their treatment also increased. In 1980 public dollars covered over three-fifths of all hospital expenditures. There was a striking increase, close to a doubling, in the number of patients cared for in nursing homes, both in skilled nursing facilities and in health-related facilities. Once again, the increase in public dollars played a crucial role; in 1980 they accounted for 66 percent of all nursing home expenditures.

For an overview of what happened in ambulatory care, it is necessary to combine services rendered by physicians in their private offices, in the ambulatory settings of hospitals, and in a wide array of other locations including community and specialized clinics and other sites such as public housing, prisons, and industrial plants.

The increase in office-based physicians and the much larger increase in hospital-based physicians over the decade and a half (see Chapter 6) laid the basis for a significant expansion of ambulatory care visits. The documented increase of ambulatory care visits to acute care hospitals and the calculated number of such visits to other clinics suggest that during this period, there was a rise of one-quarter, and possibly more, in total ambulatory care services.

Finally the large inflow of public dollars resulted also in an increased use of drugs, appliances, home health care, and other ancillary services.

From the data presented earlier, it is clear that the major consumers of these expanded services were, first, Medicare beneficiaries who were admitted more frequently, who stayed longer, and who received increasingly sophisticated treatment in hospitals. These beneficiaries also increased their use of ambulatory care services in physicians' offices, in hospital clinics and emergency rooms, and in other clinic settings.

The other major group that achieved greater access to inpatient, ambulatory, nursing home, and related health and dental care services were persons enrolled in Medicaid. In many instances, public dollars paid for services which the poor had previously received free of charge from physicians and voluntary hospitals. But the fact that

Medicaid now paid for most of these services should not obscure three critical facts: the poor had broader access to many services, particularly nursing homes, dental care and drugs; they were able to obtain more services than previously; and they had a broader choice of providers.

What happened to the 700,000 near-poor, who were never eligible for Medicaid or who were removed after the State tightened the rules and regulations, is less clear. The large municipal health care system which had earlier provided care to all persons who sought it continued to do so after the enactment of Medicaid. And to a lesser degree, many voluntary hospitals and clinics continued to provide care free of charge or at reduced rates for low-income persons who were unable to qualify for Medicaid.

The Louis Harris survey undertaken on behalf of The Commonwealth Fund in 1982 queried a representative group of New Yorkers about their health care. The findings revealed that although a considerable number of New Yorkers, over half a million, had no form of health insurance, the vast majority (six out of seven) reported that they received all the health care they sought and seven out of ten stated they had a regular source from which they received care.

The intriguing question is what a comparable survey would have revealed in 1965. It is just possible that the proportion of the total population from which positive responses were elicited would have approximated the proportion in 1982. The reason for this surmise is that the municipal health care system, supplemented by the voluntary system, provided care for all persons who sought assistance. We are not arguing that the tremendous inflow of public dollars after 1965 did not result in more and better services; we stipulate only that higher expectations of the citizenry went hand in hand with the larger expenditures. In the earlier period, the elderly did not expect to be hospitalized and treated unless they had a life-threatening condition and not always then. And the poor did not expect that the government would pay for their care in nursing homes or at home.

This brings us to the third issue: Who provided most of the additional and more intensive services that resulted from the marked increase in public dollars? In brief, the major providers were voluntary hospitals. The number of inpatient days in municipal hospitals declined both absolutely and relatively. In nursing homes, the much increased dollar flow led to a sizable expansion in both voluntary and proprietary establishments.

The analysis of ambulatory care is more complicated and the changing roles of different groups of physicians will be considered in more detail in the next chapter. For now, the following provides an initial overview. The house staffs at both voluntary and municipal hospitals were responsible for the increased number and range of ambulatory services. There were also considerable numbers of physicians, assisted by part- and full-time allied health workers who staffed various nonhospital clinics operated largely under voluntary auspices, some financed and managed by government.

The number of physicians in private practice increased and many patients who had formerly been treated for nothing or for a modest fee in a hospital setting now received ambulatory care from these private physicians who received reimbursement from government. The same shift from free to reimbursed care occurred for many of the inpatient population. Previously, they had been cared for by the resident or visiting staff and paid little. After Medicare and Medicaid, their care was reimbursed by the government.

As we will see in Chapter 7, the large influx of new dollars made it much easier for all groups of allied health workers and for hospital service workers to renegotiate the terms of their employment and to obtain relatively large increases in wages and benefits.

The last point that warrants consideration is the impact of these large public dollar expenditures for health care on the governmental funders and providers. We noted earlier the steep rise in the tax levy funds that New York City had to raise. And the pressure continued on municipal government even after improved billing by the Health and Hospitals Corporation in the early 1980s removed some of the pressures. But while these larger revenues eased the pressure on the operating budget, they did little on the capital front. The long-term shortage of capital funds has led to the continuing erosion of the plant and equipment of a substantial portion of the municipal hospital system, the greatest deficiencies being at Kings County and Queens Hospital Center.

The State found it necessary not only to prune the Medicaid rolls and to cut back on services, but also to cap its payments to physicians and hospitals for inpatient and ambulatory care. Despite these moves, the State was under continuing financial pressures which contributed to its promulgating a year-long moratorium (1983) on requests for capital construction because approval of proposed certificate of need applications would add $150 million annually to its Medicaid bill.

In absolute and relative terms, the contribution of the federal government to health care expenditures in New York City outpaced all other payers. From a base of $133 million in 1966, its total outlays in 1983 amounted to $3.7 billion.

The National Health Policy Forum, a group based in Washington, D.C., reported after a field visit to New York City in mid–1982 and in a later update: "A dominant theme in New York and for the health industry as a whole is the scarcity of money relative to the enormity of unmet need." The only reasonable conclusion from the preceding analysis is that New York City did not suffer from a "scarcity of money" and the Harris poll failed to reveal any enormous current unmet needs.

6

Physicians

Among the most important effects of the enlarged dollar flow into the health care system was its impact on physicians and other personnel who deliver health care. For it is professionals, and in the final analysis the physicians, who are responsible for overseeing most of the services that are subsumed under the category of "health care." Conventional wisdom holds that physicians determine between 70 and 80 percent of all expenditures for health care. Accordingly, this chapter will examine some of the important effects of the inflows of the new dollars on the numbers, practice modes, and work loads of the principal groups of physicians who practiced in New York City prior to the introduction of Medicare and Medicaid. We will also review the changes that occurred in physicians' profiles in the decade and a half following the establishment of the new entitlement programs. The following chapter will look at nonphysician personnel employed in the health care system.

First, we will describe briefly the distinctive characteristics which have tended to differentiate the City from the rest of the country with respect to both medical practice and practitioners, particularly their education and training and their modes of practice. In addition, we will review certain demographic and economic trends that altered the texture of the urban environment during the last two decades.

New York City, Philadelphia, and Chicago are among the principal centers of American medical education. New York City was the base for six medical schools until 1963 when Mt. Sinai Hospital expanded its educational mission to become the seventh academic health center. In the mid–1970s, New York Medical College, which had been acquired by the Archdiocese of New York in 1978, transferred most of its academic activities to Valhalla in neighboring Westchester County although it continued its close affiliations with several hospitals in the

City for both undergraduate and graduate clinical training. In 1958–1959, the six medical schools had a total enrollment of 2,738. A decade later the figure stood at 3,033. And in 1978–1979 with the Mt. Sinai Medical School fully functioning, the total stood at 4,505, an increase of just under two-thirds in the twenty-year period.

There is only a loose connection between the location of the medical school that a student attends and where he will eventually practice. A 1975 analysis revealed that of all graduates of the New York City medical schools in practice at that time, about two-fifths were practicing in New York State. Physicians are more likely to establish a practice in the same general locality in which they pursue their graduate medical education. One of the important reasons that New York City has had a better than average ratio of physicians to population has been the disproportionate amount of residency training provided by its academic health centers, its strong voluntary teaching hospitals, its large municipal hospital system, and the considerable number of other teaching hospitals.

A report by the State Health Manpower Policy Advisory Council provides comparative data about the important role that hospitals in New York City play in graduate medical education.[1] The teaching hospitals in New York City have an average of 114 residents. The only comparable city is Boston with 104 residents per hospital. The number of residents per hospital in other major cities such as Chicago, Los Angeles, and Detroit ranges from 35 to 55.

In the tables appended to his presentation in the Proceedings of the Health Policy Forum,[2] Herbert Klarman presented interesting data about changes in house staffs in New York City and in the United States over the preceding four decades (1935 to 1978).

In 1935, when graduate education was just beginning to expand, there were 9,600 house officers in the United States of whom New York City accounted for 1,760 or over 18 percent. In 1978, the comparable figures were 58,300 and 7,300, and New York City's share had dropped to 12.5 percent.

In the 1920s and particularly in the 1930s, restrictive policies of the U.S. medical schools limited the admission of applicants from religious and ethnic minorities. And these minorities—Jewish, Irish, Italian—accounted for the majority of New York City's population. Many well-qualified Jewish candidates realized that their only prospect of becoming physicians was to pursue a medical education abroad. In the mid- and late 1930s, when Hitler precipitated the emigration from Europe of large numbers of Jewish professionals including physicians, New York City received a large inflow of physicians trained abroad. The licensing authorities in New York State had to respond to the political pressures in the City, and most of these foreign-trained physicians eventually passed their examinations and entered practice.

During the early postwar decades, prior to the introduction of Medicare and Medicaid, there was a substantial expansion of house staff positions in response to diverse factors including: the trend towards specialization in medicine; the desire of graduates of foreign medical schools to pursue graduate education in the United States which was providing sophisticated medical care; the ambitions of the chiefs of residency training; the growing awareness of many hospital administrators that they would lose out in the competitive race unless they intensified their graduate programs; and the reimbursement by selected government programs, and particularly by Blue Cross and commercial insurance, to cover the direct costs of training residents as well as the costs of supervisory staff physicians.

Because of the relatively slow pace of expansion by U.S. medical schools in the 1950s and early 1960s—federal dollars did not become available for medical education until 1963—there were roughly two house staff positions available for each U.S. graduate. The reform of the immigration laws in 1965 made it much easier for foreign physicians to be admitted to the United States to pursue residency training. In 1975, of the 8,400 house staff in New York City hospitals, 4,550 were foreign medical graduates (FMGs), primarily aliens but including a significant number of U.S. citizens who had pursued their medical education abroad.

There are several reasons for concern about the disproportionately large number of FMGs on house staffs as well as among practicing physicians in New York City. Informed opinion holds that especially since the revision of the immigration laws in the mid–1960s which enabled large numbers of graduates from Asia to pursue their graduate medical studies in this country, the basic medical training of FMGs has been far below that of graduates of U.S. medical schools. Furthermore, a significant proportion of FMGs are not fluent in English, a major barrier to any effective communication with their English-speaking patients.

Moreover, FMGs are heavily concentrated in hospitals that are not major teaching institutions where they account for the majority of house staff. A recent analysis of the thirteen hospitals affiliated with Downstate Medical School in Brooklyn revealed the following distribution: of the 1,283 residents (exclusive of those in the State University Hospital), only one-third were graduates of U.S. medical schools; another 21 percent were US-FMGs (U.S. citizens) and 45 percent were FMGs. Of the 290 fellows at Downstate, over three-fifths were FMGs and another 11 percent US-FMGs.

New to the country, working hard to master the language and to pass their residency and licensing examinations, many FMGs gravitate to the periphery of the health care system. They are willing to accept positions that most U.S. graduates shun. This has helped many public and private institutions to obtain needed staff. On the other side, however, many of these FMGs provide an indifferent quality of care.

In addition to the unique role that FMGs have played since the 1930s and particularly in the post–World War II era in adding to the physician supply in New York City, the practice of medicine has also been affected by large-scale demographic and economic changes experienced by the City. An initial factor was the decline in the 1970s in the City's overall population of about 10 percent. Next was the out-migration in both the 1960s and the 1970s of middle-class whites from all the boroughs other than Staten Island, particularly from the Bronx and Brooklyn, and their replacement by blacks and Hispanics. Many physicians who were in their early or middle years of practice pulled up stakes shortly before or after their patients left and relocated in the suburbs. New graduates were understandably disinclined to open a practice in a deteriorating neighborhood not only because of the shrinking base of paying patients but also because of the lack of security for life and property. The relatively low ceiling that the State placed and maintained on reimbursements for Medicaid patients acted as a further deterrent to the survival of private practice in low-income areas.

Data about the number of physicians, the number in active practice, the type of practice, hours of work, hospital affiliations, earnings, and other critical information are not collected systematically or routinely and are not published by any agency although state licensing authorities and the American Medical Association are major repositories of some of this information. From time to time, states conduct special one-time surveys. The figures used in the following analysis are therefore first approximations, nothing more.

In the decade following the introduction of Medicare and Medicaid the total number of nonfederal physicians in New York City increased relatively modestly from 23,110 to 25,000. The increase in the number of physicians engaged part-time or full-time in patient care was considerably smaller, from 20,800 to 21,400. If we consider only physicians who are involved exclusively in patient care and who are not hospital based, the number ranges from 11,300 to 13,300; this was foreshadowed by our earlier discussion of neighborhood change.

Of course, the foregoing changes must be placed in the context of a declining City population which dropped from 7.9 million in 1970 to 7.1 million in 1980. It is also necessary to consider the distribution of physicians in the five boroughs. According to the responses to the

State Department of Education's survey of licensed physicians in the City in 1980–1981,[3] there were 20,496 of whom 18,546 returned usable questionnaires. Although Manhattan accounted for under 20 percent of the City's population in 1980, half of the physicians worked there; this resulted in a ratio of one licensed physician for every 135 persons. In contrast the ratios for the other three large boroughs were: for the Bronx, 1:633; for Brooklyn, 1:618; and for Queens, 1:514. Even after allowance is made for the fact that many residents of the other boroughs seek medical care in Manhattan, particularly specialist care, the distribution is skewed.

The increasing numbers of blacks and Hispanics in the population indicates that we should look more closely at the number and the distribution of minority physicians who practice in the City. According to the aforementioned survey, of the approximately 18,500 respondents only 579 were black and 375 were Hispanic. By far the largest minority group consisted of Asian physicians who numbered 2,380.

At the time of this survey, New York City had 1.8 million blacks and 1.4 million Hispanics, and Manhattan contained 17 percent of the black and 24 percent of the Hispanic population. It accounted, however, for the practice locations of 45 percent of both the black and Hispanic physicians.

Of the 18,546 surveyed physicians, Table 6.1 shows the following concentrations of specialties:

Only in pediatrics was Manhattan's share below 40 percent. In all of the other major specialties Manhattan accounted for half and in some fields, such as surgery, considerably more than half. In only two small specialties, emergency medicine and family practice, did Manhattan have less than its proportionate share.

In the mid–1970s, based on an analysis of the American Medical Association master file, the distribution of physicians in New York City revealed the following: just under half of all physicians (49 percent) were in nonhospital-based patient care; just under one-third were residents; and the remainder were equally divided between full-time hospital staff and those engaged in nonpatient care activity, primarily education, research, and administration.

During the decade, all of the boroughs experienced an increase in the physician–population ratio, with Manhattan showing the biggest gain, 28 percent, and the Bronx the smallest gain, 8 percent.

Simultaneously with this period of expansion, both the Bronx and Brooklyn experienced significant declines in the ratios of nonhospital-based physicians engaged in patient care to population; they lost one-quarter and one-fifth respectively. In 1976, the Bronx had only 73 nonhospital-based physicians per 100,000 population while the ratio for Manhattan was more than fivefold greater (398 per 100,000).

Table 6.1 Concentration of Physician Specialties, New York City, 1980–1981

Internal Medicine	4,484
Psychiatry, Neurology	2,735
Pediatrics	1,535
Surgery	1,089
Obstetrics, Gynecology	1,073
Orthopedic Surgery	911
General Practice	887
Radiology	737
Family Practice	684

The United Hospital Fund has developed a table (6.2) which provides additional information about the changes in the field of practice of office-based physicians during the 1970s:

In a period when the city-wide ratio of office-based physicians increased by roughly 15 percent, the proportion of physicians in general practice declined by more than two-fifths. In 1970, New York City was slightly above the U.S. average for physicians in general practice but by the decade's end it stood at 25 percent below the national average which had declined from 25 to 21, compared with the City's which fell from 28 to 16.

We are now in a better position to identify at least some of the impacts of the increased flow of health care dollars on the number and characteristics of the physicians and their practice profiles.

The initial impetus to expand both undergraduate and graduate medical education in New York City was well under way prior to the passage of Medicare and Medicaid. It had been supported in funding by the State, research grants from the National Institutes of Health, third-party reimbursement for the extra costs of residency training, and increased contributions by philanthropy. But the major increases in residency training followed the introduction of Medicare and Medicaid. Reimbursement for their beneficiaries assured that hospitals could recapture most of the costs involved in developing larger and more elaborate graduate training programs, including more substantial stipends for residents and fellows. The early increases in expenditures for patient care became the foundation for an expansion of graduate and even undergraduate medical education because of the role that residents play in instructing undergraduates during their clerkships.

The new dollars for patient care covered not only the salaries of the residents but also enabled most large and many smaller hospitals to

Physicians

Table 6.2 Field of Practice, Office–based Physicians, New York City, 1970, 1975, and 1980

	Per 100,000 Population		
Field	1970	1975	1980
General Practice	28	21	16
Medical Specialties	43	46	59
Surgical Specialties	39	37	44
Other Specialties	34	35	46
Total	144	139	165

add full-time supervisory staff to oversee and direct the residency programs. The several specialty societies accredit residency programs on the basis of whether they have a sufficiently large and varied inflow of patients to provide broad clinical experience for those in training, the qualifications of the teaching staff including the presence of a full-time senior physician to direct the program, the adequacy of equipment and space, and the breadth, depth, and integration of the successive stages in the learning process.

In the early 1960s, there was a sharp jump in the salaries paid to interns and residents. By 1963, interns in municipal hospitals earned $175 per month up from $105 per month in 1957.

Once the financial position of the hospitals began to ease as a result of more reimbursement by third-party payers, interns and residents began to press for substantial improvements in pay and fringe benefits as well as reductions in their hours on duty and the time that they were on call. They made significant gains, usually without having to resort to strike action. In 1975, however, a strike was called in twenty-one voluntary hospitals and as a result, the residents made additional gains. In contrast, the strike that was called in the municipal hospital system in 1981 which was directed primarily to forcing the New York City Health and Hospitals Corporation to improve the quality of patient care petered out without any significant gains to the strikers. The use of the strike tactic to impel reform and improvement in the conditions of patient care failed to elicit broad rank and file support and failed almost completely to arouse public support since both the politicians and the press looked upon the strike as the wrong instrument to accomplish the desired goals.

The enlarged inflow of patient care money into the health care system increased the opportunities for residents to supplement their hospital stipends by taking part-time assignments on their own time. Although this type of moonlighting was frowned upon, the practice grew in the post–World War II era when residents were no longer required to live on hospital premises and were assigned to more or less regular shifts.

The United Hospital Fund's study of hospital manpower for 1978[4] provides some telling details about the direct dollar outlays for graduate medical education. In its summary data for seventy-six voluntary and proprietary hospitals and one state hospital (Downstate University Hospital), total expenses came to $2.8 billion, of which salaries amounted to $1.6 billion. These hospitals employed a total of 5,683 residents and interns with an average annual salary (exclusive of fringe benefits) of $17,000 and 2,480 supervisory physicians with an annual average salary of $30,000. In addition, there were 381 physicians in nonapproved residency training programs.

The salaries for residents amounted to 5.9 percent of all salaries, those for supervisory physicians to 4.6 percent and another 0.6 percent for physicians in nonapproved programs; together, they constituted 11.1 percent of total salaries. Translated into dollars, the direct costs of training residents in 1978 in New York City came to $181 million. Since the overwhelming proportion of all residency training was concentrated in voluntary hospitals (and selected municipal hospitals which were not included in the survey), the more relevant data relate to the fifty-nine voluntary hospitals whose combined salaries for residents and supervisory physicians came to 11.4 percent of a total salary expense of $1.5 billion or just under $175 million.

Some additional information can be extracted from the hospitals in Blue Cross Groups I, II, and III which together paid for most of the residents' salaries—4,223 out of a total of 5,683 residents, or just under three-quarters. The average salaries of the residents amounted to $16,000 for Group I, $19,000 for Group II, and $17,300 for Group III, which suggests that the most prestigious academic health center hospitals were able to compete successfully even though they offered somewhat lower salaries. The salaries they paid supervisory physicians were likewise lower: Group I, $27,700 compared to $33,500 in Group II, and $29,400 in Group III.

The most striking finding is that the few large teaching hospitals in Group II spent 15.5 percent of their total salaries of $332 million on residents and supervisory physicians, far more than Group I and Group III hospitals whose outlays for these salaries came to 10.9 and 12.9 percent respectively. Once again it could be inferred that greater effort was required of Group II hospitals to pace the leaders.

It would be a mistake, however, to assess the total costs of residency training in terms of direct outlays for salaries to residents and supervisory physicians. There are important indirect costs associated with extensive teaching programs that stem from the more elaborate use of diagnostic and therapeutic procedures, differential patient mix, and a longer patient stay. The United Hospital Fund study reveals the following differences in salary expense per patient-day among hospitals in the three largest groups: $194 for Group I hospitals, $185 for Group II, and $159 for Group III.

The foregoing suggests that large training programs add significantly to the costs of operating a hospital. However, a more reasonable formulation might be that large training programs alter both the inputs and the outputs of hospitals that sponsor them. Before World War II, when only a relatively small proportion of all medical graduates continued their studies beyond internship (today called the first year of residency), most medium-size and large hospitals in New York City relied on volunteer physicians to take care of clinic patients and inpatients who were unable to pay or who could pay only part of their bill. At academic health centers, the members of the medical school faculty interested in clinical medicine devoted a considerable number of hours each week to the care of the indigent.

The increase in sophisticated technology together with the trend toward specialization that marked the post–World War II decades filled the acute hospitals with sicker patients who required more sophisticated services. The declining reliance on voluntary staff and the greater reliance on salaried interns and residents represented adaptations to the changing therapeutic environment of the hospital which also dovetailed with the need for expanded teaching programs. The hospital staff, rather than the admitting physician, was better able to provide continuing oversight of patients, many of whom required close supervision and frequent therapeutic interventions. The voluntary staff also benefited from the large number of ambitious house staff who wanted to hone their skills by undertaking much of the preparatory and follow-up procedures for the patients who were admitted for surgery or for medical diagnosis and therapy.

Hospitals with large numbers of residents were also in a better position to expand their emergency rooms and clinics in response to the growing needs of patients who sought care in their outpatient departments because of the decline in private practitioners in their neighborhoods.

Since board certified specialists were finding it relatively easy to obtain hospital appointments, since many younger physicians were opening practices in the suburbs, and since the number of general practitioners remaining in the City was declining, hospitals with large ambulatory care services were no longer able to rely primarily on volunteers to staff their clinics and their burgeoning emergency rooms. Residents filled these expanding areas, and hospitals without adequate house staff had to hire salaried physicians to provide part or all of the medical care.

The willingness of Medicare and Medicaid to reimburse hospitals for the ambulatory care services they provided represented a new source of funds. Blue Cross also took a series of halting steps to broaden its reimbursement policies for outpatient care for services that were considered an alternative to inpatient treatment. Blue Cross eventually introduced an additional reimbursement factor (community service) to assist voluntary hospitals which provided much free or below-cost outpatient care.

Because of the complexity of hospital cost accounting which involves the allocation of joint services between inpatients and outpatients, it is impossible for an outsider to assess whether a reimbursement rate of $60 for an emergency room visit for a Medicaid patient is too low or whether a Medicare rate of $80 or even $90 is adequate. What is not subject to dispute is the large number of ambulatory patients whom hospitals treat who have no coverage and who are able to pay little, if any of the total charge for their care. Large teaching hospitals with extensive ambulatory care programs believe that their low operating margins reflect the large amount of unrequited services that they provide.

The analysis up to this point suggests that the increased dollar flows had the following impacts on physicians and their practice modes: a marked decline in the number of physicians providing voluntary inpatient and outpatient care for the City's indigent; a transformation of the staffs of teaching hospitals as the result of the appointment of large numbers of salaried physicians overseeing training programs, and the still larger numbers of residents (and fellows) enrolled in graduate medical programs; the financial support of Blue Cross, Medicare, Medicaid, and private insurance for this expanded staff and for other costs of graduate medical education; changes in the control and treatment of both inpatients and outpatients with residents, under supervision, assuming greater responsibility; and the critical role that residents came to play in the provision of health care especially in two large boroughs—Bronx and Brooklyn—with their growing numbers of minorities.

In the mid–1970s, residents accounted for a high proportion of all primary care providers in these two boroughs. In the Bronx, residents accounted for between 50 and 60 percent of all internists, pediatricians, and general surgeons, and for more than two-fifths of all obstetricians and gynecologists. Put the other way, less than 30 percent of all internists, pediatricians and surgeons were engaged in nonhospital-based patient care.

The figures for Brooklyn are slightly less extreme but even there residents provided close to half of all primary care and, with the single exception of obstetrics/gynecology, less than 40 percent of all active physicians in primary care were not among hospital-based staff.

Two further points should be noted. At the end of the 1970s about half of all residents were FMGs or US-FMGs and a disproportionate number of them were concentrated in hospitals caring for patients in the outer boroughs (other than Manhattan). Reformulated, it follows that a significant proportion of all minority and low-income persons who obtained their ambulatory and inpatient care from voluntary and municipal hospitals in the Bronx and Brooklyn were being treated by foreigners who had graduated from foreign medical schools.

The same combination of foreign birth and foreign medical education also characterized the majority of physicians who provided care in the 350 "shared health facilities." These were the so-called Medicaid mills. It was estimated in the mid–1970s that these facilities billed for about $200 million of Medicaid reimbursement annually. It is clear that the patients they treated could not be considered to be in the mainstream of U.S. medicine.

Another consequence of the changing structure of care for inpatients and outpatients supported by the enlarged reimbursement flows from third-party payers was the opportunity it offered for a significant proportion of physicians to combine fee-for-service medicine with a part- or full-time salaried position. Earlier reference was made to the fact that in 1978, supervisory physicians in the major teaching hospitals received on the average between $27,000 and $33,000 as salary from the employing hospital. Most physicians with salaried appointments are permitted to earn stipulated amounts above their salaries. At Downstate Medical Center, gross violations of the State's stipulated ceilings for "outside" earnings have been reported from time to time.

In recent years when the total dollars flowing into the health care system have become more constrained, the major academic health centers—and their principal affiliates—have established and expanded physician practice plans whereby members of the clinical faculty must contribute some proportion of their earnings—ranging from 15 to 30 percent—to a fund, part of which is remitted to the dean, part to their department for research or to other special projects such as the support of additional fellows.

One of the striking impacts of the expanded hospital reimbursements, particularly reimbursements from Medicare, was the ability of physicians to charge for many services which they had previously provided free to both inpatients and ambulatory patients. Since the reimbursement schedules favored physicians who made extensive use of procedures, particularly surgeons, their previously comfortable earnings level was usually raised a notch or two. If a physician had formerly devoted the equivalent of one or one-and-a-half days out of a five-and-a-half-day week to work for which he previously received no fees, the new reimbursement arrangements implied a gain of between 25 and 30 percent in his annual income. But that understates the impact of the new reimbursement system because physicians' fees geared to the "usual, customary, and reasonable" criterion advanced more rapidly than the CPI.

Reliable data on physicians' incomes are difficult, some would say impossible, to come by. Most surveys rely on self-reporting. Moreover, perspective over longer periods of time requires that one consider not only gross earnings but also changes in the costs of running a practice. In New York City, the variations around the average have been pronounced with the top-earning specialists having billings of five to ten times those of the average practitioner.

In the year that Medicare and Medicaid were passed, an analysis based on income tax returns revealed that physicians, exclusive of house staff, in the New York–Standard Metropolitan Statistical Area (NY–SMSA), that is, the City proper plus the immediately surrounding suburbs, had average annual earnings of $20,000; salaried physicians earned about $4,000 less, and physicians in private practice earned about $3,000 more. Only anesthesiologists earned more than an average of $30,000 and four other specialties yielded average earnings between $25,000 and $30,000; in descending order they were surgery, obstetrics/gynecology, psychiatry, and radiology. In 1965 the mean for the NY–SMSA was about 16 percent below those of other SMSAs, and the earnings of self-employed physicians in the New York area was the second lowest of the twenty-five SMSAs included in the study. In fact, the poor showing of New York reflected the high proportion of salaried physicians, in excess of 36 percent.

In 1976, the total number of physicians in New York City was estimated at just under 25,000, of whom 18,700 were engaged primarily in patient care. Of these, about 10,000 were office-based and the remainder were hospital-based. The State Education Department's survey for 1980–1981 suggests that the numbers did not change much in the ensuing four years after we add to the 22,000 licensed physicians about half of the 8,000 residents (who are not licensed), yielding a total figure of around 26,000.

There is no firm basis for estimating what happened to physicians' incomes in New York City in the decade and a half after Medicare and Medicaid; nor would a single figure be particularly revealing. The presumption is that because of the large number of salaried physicians, including the large number of residents, the finding of the mid–1960s would continue to hold—the average earnings of physicians in New York City would probably be below the average for most other metropolitan areas by some 10 or 15 percent.

The following issues must be taken into account in assessing the likely changes that occurred among different subgroups of physicians during the period when the dollar inflows increased substantially. To start at the bottom: residents made significant gains in terms of higher stipends and reduced schedules which in turn enabled many of them to moonlight and thereby increase their earnings substantially. On the other hand, when they had completed their graduate medical education, most of them did not find the City a conducive environment in which to start a full-time practice. Costs of office practice had risen considerably as a result of steep increases in malpractice insurance, rents (in Manhattan), and the salary levels for office personnel. The best prospect for newly minted specialists was to combine an institutional appointment at a medical school and/or a major teaching hospital with a split form of private practice, part in the suburbs and part at the medical center in the City. Many followed this pattern. Others left the City to practice in other areas, near and far.

The large number of salaried physicians, especially those attached to medical schools who had earlier been devoting most or all of their time to education and research, have come under increasing pressure in recent years with the leveling off and decline in National Institutes of Health dollars to earn at least part of their salary through patient care.

The senior clinicians attached to academic health centers and to major teaching hospitals have also come under increasing pressure in recent years to join practice plans which assure that some part of their fees becomes available to meet the increasingly straitened budgets of their institutions. Some of the highest earners, those with loose academic ties, have refused to be taxed and have resigned their clinical professorships rather than join the practice plans.

The established specialists with affiliations to a strong teaching hospital, except for those in pediatrics, psychiatry, and obstetrics/gynecology, have generally done well over the intervening period because of the increased volume of ambulatory and inpatient care which has been reimbursed by Medicare and the large numbers of other patients with broad insurance coverage. The costs of private practice have increased substantially but most established specialists have been able to stay ahead, particularly if their hospital covers part or all of the costs of their malpractice insurance.

As the earlier figures revealed, the number of office-based general practitioners and specialists providing primary care has been declining. Those located in impoverished neighborhoods have not fared well. Some have retired early and others have shifted into salaried positions, often administrative.

In completing this broad assessment of the impact of the new dollar flows on physicians' earnings we must take note of the changes in work schedules. Based on replies from respondents in the entire State of New York, the Physician Manpower Survey for 1980–1981 contains the interesting finding that only about one-third of all physicians devoted more than 40 hours a week to professional activities and about two out of five spent between 30 and 40 hours. The remainder spent less time which suggests that they were not engaged full-time in the practice of medicine. These data, when placed alongside earlier surveys, strongly suggest that one of the important gains that most physicians made over the past two decades has been the reduction in the length of their workday, workweek, and work year.

7

The Unionization of Health Care Workers

Physicians are the leaders of the health care team; they make most of the decisions relating to diagnosis and therapy. But physicians cannot perform without the assistance of many others, professionals and nonprofessionals, who undertake important functions in the care of patients, ambulatory and bedridden. At the turn of this century, physicians accounted for about one in every three health care workers; nurses, most of whom had little formal training, were the next largest group. Today, depending on how we define the health care industry and how we classify health care employees, each of the approximately 450,000 physicians is supported by between 13 and 16 other workers.

An analysis that seeks to trace the impact of the increased dollar flows on the health care system must therefore consider the employment and earnings of nonphysician health workers. Since the data relating to the numbers and earnings of health care workers attached to institutions, particularly hospitals and nursing homes, are more detailed and reliable than for those employed by private practitioners, independent clinics, and similar types of establishments, the following analysis will focus on the hospital sector which, we must remember, provides employment for about 70 percent of all nonprofessional health care workers. We will concentrate on the largest groups: nursing personnel, workers in housekeeping and property maintenance, administrative personnel, and nutrition and food service workers who in total account for about three-quarters of the hospital's work force.

Until the end of World War II, hospital employment differed considerably from employment in the competitive market; thereafter, hospitals required considerable time to become fully integrated into the market system. Therefore, we will recall briefly some of the characteristics that governed hospital employment in past decades.

Most general care hospitals were under nonprofit or government auspices and as such offered their employees more job security than wages. Unless his performance was egregious, a hospital employee could expect to hold his or her job indefinitely. Since philanthropy played a role in the support of many hospitals, it was assumed that not only the physicians who spent time caring for poor patients free of charge but all hospital staff placed less importance on monetary rewards than on the privilege of being able to help their fellows in times of sickness or injury. Some of the rewards of the hospital staff were free meals, medical care for themselves and occasionally for members of their families, and the absence of pressure to achieve and maintain a high level of output per hour of work. The National Labor Relations Act of 1938 specifically exempted nonprofit (and government) institutions such as hospitals from its provisions which meant that if the hospital work force attempted to organize to improve its wages and conditions of work, it could not look for assistance from the Board.

The other major characteristics of the hospital sector that warrant brief note are the following: the predominance of female workers, above 75 percent; the large number of minority workers in low paying jobs; the shift in nursing education after World War II out of the hospital into collegiate settings; the high proportion of all hospital jobs that had few formal educational or other requirements; and the barriers to upward mobility across occupational categories.

According to a late 1960 study of the municipal hospitals in New York City, only one in every four positions required preparation beyond a high school diploma and over two-thirds did not require a diploma. Put baldly, we can say that most hospitals followed the practice of recruiting most of their nonprofessional personnel from among the unskilled members of the work force.

Between 1960 and 1977, health employees in nongovernment institutions increased in New York City from 97,000 to 184,500. In 1966 the number stood at about 118,000—up 21,000 over the preceding six years. In the six years following Medicare and Medicaid (1966–1972), the total reached 156,400, an increase of over 38,000. The next year 1973, saw the largest increase—18,000 additional employees or a gain of close to 12 percent. It was followed by the gain of another 6,000 in 1974; the total rose from 174,000 to 180,000, after which it leveled off at 184,000 for the next three years.

The public sector trends are somewhat different. The municipal hospitals increased their health personnel from 38,600 in 1961 to about 47,000 in 1975 or by 22 percent, a more modest rate of increase than among voluntary and proprietary hospitals. Most of the increases were made after 1970. In terms of municipal service employment overall, hospitals had the third lowest rate of increase. Moreover, in absolute numbers the hospital sector lagged behind education, welfare and higher education which had increases of 24,000, 18,000 and 15,000, respectively, between the early 1960s and the mid–1970s.

The impressive overall growth of health services employment in New York was consistent with national trends. Between 1960 and 1977, the total number of health employees in the United States increased from about 1.5 million to close to 4.6 million, or by more than threefold. Only once (1973) in these seventeen years did the rate of increase in New York City exceed that for the country as a whole.

Our special study of twenty-four hospitals for the period 1966–1976 showed a notably slower rate of increase in employment, 37 percent versus 57 percent for all health personnel in nongovernment institutions. However, we can extract several interesting insights from this special sample. The largest hospitals, Blue Cross Groups I through IV had increases of between 34 and 41 percent while the smaller and specialty hospitals experienced increases ranging only from 9 to 20 percent.

The nursing area claimed the largest number of new employees, about 11,400 out of 36,400 but in terms of percentages, the nursing staff grew by only 14 percent. Household personnel likewise had a much below average rate of increase, amounting to 15 percent although it represented the second largest absolute category, accounting for 7,200 additional employees. Only one segment of the sample, hospitals in Group III, were able to get through the decade with very little increase (2 percent) in household personnel. If we were to speculate why this was so, we might say that it reflects two conditions: a more modern plant and less need for security guards.

The third functional area relates to administrative personnel which increased over the decade an average of 46 percent. Proprietary hospitals were able to hold the line and added on the average only one person to their administrative rolls. Group III and Group IV hospitals had increases far above the average, amounting to 66 and 89 percent respectively. It may be that when the exceptionally large gains in Group IV are juxtaposed to the stability in its household personnel, there may be overlapping between the two functions.

The only other observation we will add about the expansion of employment during the two decades refers to the growth that took place in the capacity and utilization of nursing homes where the work force expanded to accommodate the large expansion in beds.

The foregoing data indicate that one impact of the new dollars flowing into the health care system was the expansion of the size of the work force which was linked to the larger numbers of hospital admissions and more intensified treatment as well as to an expansion of ambulatory and nursing home care.

The more dramatic impact of additional dollars on the health care work force was the changes in wages, fringe benefits, work rules, and hours of work, all of which were strikingly altered in the quarter century between the late 1950s and the mid–1980s. A critical factor in the changes that occurred was the organization of workers into two major trade unions and several smaller ones. District Council 37 of the American Federation of State, County and Municipal Employees (AFSCME) gained control over the nonprofessional health care staff in the municipal hospitals, and Local 1199 of the Drug and Hospital Workers Union came to represent most workers in the voluntary hospital sector. Early in the history of union activity among health care workers in the municipal system, Local 237 of the Teamsters had the inside track but it lost out to District Council 37. Reference should also be made to Local 144 of the Hotel and Allied Services Union which tried to enroll members from among the personnel of proprietary hospitals. Finally, Local 302 of AFSCME competed with Local 1199 in efforts to organize employees of selected voluntary hospitals. When the smoke cleared, District Council 37 and Local 1199 emerged as the two dominant unions, but the period of conflict between the unions and the employing hospitals and among the unions themselves lasted for the better part of fifteen years, from the late 1950s until the early 1970s.

The dynamic improvements in the wages and working conditions of the lowest rung of hospital employees, the unskilled workers employed in housekeeping functions, can best be appreciated by considering the terms of their employment as late as 1958. In that year, those at the bottom of the hospital hierarchy earned between $28 and $30 for a 44- to 48-hour week, often stretched over six working days. While comparisons across occupational and industry categories are difficult, it is noteworthy that in 1960 average weekly earnings of production workers in New York City (predominantly low-wage industries) amounted to $85 for a 40-hour week. We can acknowledge that an operative in the garment industry had more skill and potential than a member of a hospital's housekeeping staff; nevertheless, the gap would not justify a differential of 200 percent in wages and between 10 and 20 percent in working hours. These differences reflected other factors, of course, including an ample supply of unskilled workers and the absence of trade unions.

Montefiore broke ranks with the voluntary hospitals and signed with Local 1199 in the late 1950s but only after applying successful pressure on the City to raise its reimbursement rates for welfare patients. This three-cornered relationship—involving trade unions pressuring for improved contracts, the hospitals holding the line, and City and later State government controlling the purse via reimbursements—set the stage for most of the ensuing employee/employer bargaining, particularly after the State statutes (1963) and later the federal statutes (1974) were amended to entitle workers in voluntary hospitals to organize and seek collective bargaining agreements. The other critical development was the passage of Medicare and Medicaid in 1965, and their reimbursement rates which expanded the opportunities for hospitals to cover their rising costs.

In 1958, when the employees of Montefiore Hospital were organized, minimum wages were in the range of $34–$38 per week. The new contract established a minimum of $40 a week and stipulated a basic work week of 40 hours after which time and a half would be paid (and not, as previously, compensated by time off or straight time). Valuable fringe benefits were established including 10 days sick leave which could be accumulated up to 30 days, as well as a grievance procedure. Mayor Wagner promised that the City would aim to double its reimbursement rate for welfare clients from $10 to $20 per day to help Montefiore meet the more than half million dollar increase in its wage bill over the two-year contract.

At the time when Montefiore signed with Local 1199, the City had a minimum weekly wage of $53 for its employees which led Barry Feinstein, the head of the Teamsters local, to accuse Leon Davis, president of Local 1199, of entering into a "sweetheart" contract with Montefiore Hospital.

In the late 1950s, Mayor Wagner's administration had taken two steps which gave an edge to City employees. Most of them were included in a classification system which enabled them to obtain periodic wage increases. And the mayor was moving, in advance of the governor, to permit the organization of City employees into trade unions of their own choosing.

As the following data make clear, hospital employees in New York City made larger gains than hospital employees in other parts of the country in the years immediately preceding the introduction of Medicare and Medicaid (Table 7.1). These gains reflected a combination of circumstances: the most important were the initiative of both the City and the State in facilitating the organization of hospital employees, the improvements in the wage scale for municipal employees, strong initiatives by professional nursing organizations, and an increasingly tight labor market. The impact of these several favorable forces can be read in the comparisons for the years 1963–1966 in Table 7.1.

Equally striking were the differentially greater gains among hospi-

Table 7.1   Rates of Wage Increase for Hospital Employees, 1963–1966
(in percent)

Employee	New York City	United States
Licensed practical nurse	19.5%	5.7%
Nursing aide	8.0	1.7
Kitchen worker	19.1	5.9
Maid	17.5	2.9
Porter	17.5	8.7
Switchboard operator	12.3	5.1
Transcribing machine operator	6.0	2.0

tal employees. Licensed practical nurses, for example, achieved increases of 19 percent while their colleagues in other parts of the United States increased their wages 6 percent. Other hospital employees in New York City were also able to begin to close the gap that had existed between them and other skilled and unskilled service-workers. For instance, in New York City the wages of hospital kitchen workers increased 19 percent while secretaries averaged only a 7 percent gain during these years.

In the three years after the passage of Medicare and Medicaid both nonprofessional workers and registered nurses in New York City continued to make gains of the same magnitude as they had in the immediately preceding period, mostly in the 15–20 percent range, while secretaries averaged only a 2 percent increase.

If we look at the figures for these six crucial years before and after Medicare and Medicaid (1963–1969) in Table 7.2, we find that the rate of change was definitely in favor of health care employees and that in New York City wage increases for hospital employees outdistanced the national rate.

The success that Local 1199 achieved in organizing the voluntary hospitals in the years following 1958 reflected more than the aggressive leadership of its president, Leon Davis. The struggling union was able to elicit substantial support from the trade union leadership in the City, at least from among those unions with which it was not in competition. Furthermore, 1199 provided one of the first opportunities for blacks and Puerto Ricans to play an active role in bettering their position. The voluntary hospital establishment mistakenly assumed that the citizenry and the press would be hostile to any organizing efforts directed at hospitals and simply would not tolerate strikes. But that is not what happened. Repeatedly, important political and public figures spoke out in urging hospital trustees to sit down and try to work out a reasonable settlement with their workers who were threatening to strike or who were already on the picket lines.

The trustees who sought to pit the poorly paid employees against

Table 7.2   Rates of Wage Increase for Hospital Employees, 1963–1969
(in percent)

Employee	New York City	United States
Licensed practical nurse	40%	28%
Nursing aide	22	19
Kitchen worker	40	23
Maid	37	23
Porter	36	24
Switchboard operator	25	15
Transcribing machine operator	45	13
Nurse		
Supervisor	48	32
Head	41	34
General duty	43	36

the sick and injured failed. There was broad sympathy, surely in the 1960s and even into the 1970s, among the public for the legitimacy of many of the claims that the unions were making on behalf of their members.

Ten years after its initial contract with Montefiore Hospital in July 1968, Local 1199 was able to negotiate a two-year contract with many leading voluntary hospitals which had earlier established a League of Voluntary Hospitals to improve their bargaining position. This settlement gave the workers a gain of slightly over 30 percent in wages and fringe benefits. Once again, the political leadership played a critical role. Hospital reimbursement rates were raised by $20 a day which, Mayor Lindsay remarked, represented "a fair and equitable settlement for all involved." The minimum wage was set at $100 a week and those who were earning above the minimum received a 16 percent increase or $24 per week. The union also won a contributory pension plan and a fund for training and upgrading workers.

Over the decade, District Council 37 had succeeded in absorbing many smaller competing unions which had early gained some representation among municipal hospital workers. In the early summer of 1969, Victor Gotbaum, bargaining for the municipal employees, was able to settle with the City on very favorable terms which the mayor estimated would cost the City between $60 and $70 million over the thirty months of the contract but which despite its costs, had the advantage, in the mayor's view, of raising many workers out of poverty and making them into "firm taxpayers."

When the 1968 contract ran out, the new negotiation between Local 1199 and the League of Voluntary Hospitals became acrimonious. This time, Governor Rockefeller, who had been appealed to by the League, explained that if the settlement led to costs that could not be offset by improved management, "regular procedures are available for obtaining prompt and reasonable adjustments in their (the hospitals') rates of payment from Medicare and Medicaid." The new minimum wage was set at $130 a week (a 30 percent raise) and workers earning above the minimum received a 15 percent increase the first year and 10 percent the second, with additional significant improvements in their health and welfare benefits.

In the following year, Gotbaum negotiated an excellent three-year contract for the more than 40,000 workers who were members of District Council 37. The minimum for housekeeping workers was increased from $6,000 to $7,800 and nurses aides made comparable gains from $6,100 to $7,975. The increases averaged 27.5 percent over the life of the contract and Gotbaum emphasized that it would make those workers the highest paid in their categories in the nation.

The establishment of the New York City Health and Hospitals Corporation (HHC) in 1970 brought with it a realignment of union membership. Members of Local 1199 working in municipal hospitals were to be transferred to District Council 37 and vice versa in the voluntary sector, but Davis insisted that the wages and seniority of his members be protected. Gotbaum was initially unwilling to agree to Davis's demand. As part of the involved negotiations, HHC promised Local 1199 the right to enroll the employees of North Central Bronx Hospital, adjacent to Montefiore, when it opened. After much pulling and hauling in which the intra-union dispute got entangled in new contract negotiations for 1972–1974 between Local 1199 and the League, both issues were resolved. Davis agreed to accept the arbitrator's award which amounted to a 7.5 percent increase for each of the two years of the new contract and raised the minimum to $154 a week in 1974. And the union once again won many additional attractive benefits such as the right of workers to accumulate up to 48 days of sick leave.

The bargaining in New York City was complicated by the new federal wage and price ceilings which had been put into place. The Cost of Living Council cut the 8.3 percent increase that the 33,000 workers in the voluntary hospitals had received in 1972 back to 5.5 percent but after an appeal by Local 1199, the cut was partially restored. The League took the position that any restoration would force it to seek higher reimbursement from Blue Cross and Medicaid.

The acceleration of inflation in living costs and the interference of Washington with the terms of the settlement that Local 1199 had negotiated with the League set the stage for a major confrontation in November 1973 when Davis called 30,000 workers off their jobs forcing the closure and/or cutbacks in many ambulatory and inpatient services. Davis was fined $10,000 for calling an unauthorized strike and the court threatened additional fines. Federal mediators entered the situation with the aim of narrowing and resolving the differences between Local 1199 and the League. The situation was complicated by a decision by Blue Cross not to recognize certain costs that the hospitals incurred by virtue of the strike, particularly as a result of reduced occupancy. The Cost of Living Council convened a special panel which was able to get the parties together, but the union came away with only a 6 percent increase or $9 a week, whichever was larger. Davis found a silver lining in the episode. "We showed you can't run hospitals without the people who carry bedpans, the predominantly black and Puerto Rican people. From now on we'll have to be taken seriously."

The following year District Council 37 entered into a three-year contract with the City (1973–1976) for all its employees with special provisions for each industrial and occupational group which provided for a combination of substantial wage and benefit increases.

In 1974, Local 1199 was back negotiating a two-year contract that required the intervention of the State Industrial Commissioner before it was signed. After consultation with his colleagues in Albany and with Blue Cross in New York City, the Commissioner put forward a set of proposals that brought the minimum wage in hospitals to $181 a week and the average to $210 a week, with substantial additional benefits and a denial of the League's request for the right to subcontract.

Just as Local 1199 and District Council 37 were hitting their full stride, having organized all the important voluntary and municipal hospitals in the City with the notable exception of New York Hospital and St. Vincent's which had escaped mostly because of intraunion conflict and their existing liberal wage and benefit structures, the entire collective bargaining climate became strained. The City was approaching the onset of its devastating fiscal crisis which foreshadowed the end of liberal labor settlements and also squeezed the State's budget with direct and indirect effects on what Albany would authorize by way of reimbursements for hospital care.

The City made plans to close various municipal hospitals including Gouverneur, Delafield, Morrisania, Fordham, and Sydenham. The threat of closing Sydenham brought many in the Harlem community to protest. District Council 37 insisted that if Sydenham were closed, it would result in serious job losses and Local 1199 recognized that cutbacks in Medicaid would adversely affect the voluntary system.

District Council 37 threatened to strike on May 1976 to prevent the 3,000 layoffs one month prior to the expiration of its contract, but Gotbaum who was deeply involved in efforts to rescue the City from imminent bankruptcy, realized that the City's officials were serious when they stated that there was no money for raises and that HHC's outlays would have to be reduced. A panel under State Senator Basil Patterson recommended that 842 rather than 1,450 workers be terminated and this, together with other recommendations providing for deferrals of wage increases, enabled Gotbaum to accept the negotiated settlement.

Secretary of the Treasury William Simon stated that he would not give the City the $1.1 billion loan it urgently needed unless he were assured that neither District Council 37 nor Local 1199 would receive wage increases. The League, noting the changed environment in City Hall, Albany, and Washington, decided to adopt a hard negotiating line, realizing that henceforth it would be more difficult for its hospitals to obtain higher reimbursement rates to cover more expensive contracts.

Davis, on the other hand, realized that he had a strong union in place and that his workers were falling behind because of the escalation in the cost of living. Strikes had served him well in the past and he geared up for another. In August 1976, 1199 struck thirty-three voluntary hospitals. The Health Commissioner called the strike "inhuman and barbaric" and both Governor Carey and Mayor Beame found themselves on the spot. The Mayor pointed out that the City had "no money to throw into the situation. Any solution will have to be worked out in the absence of City funds." The State Superintendent of Insurance took a line reflecting the new fiscal stringency in Albany: "The cost of health care must be controlled by the hospital and health providers and not consistently passed along to the users through ever increasing reimbursement rates and higher insurance charges."

For a time, the League refused to submit the issues to binding arbitration but the ability of the union to tighten the noose with support from staff physicians, and the fact that the Democratic Party was holding its presidential nominating convention in the City created sufficient pressure on the League to force it into arbitration.

With money tighter, the arbitrator decided that there would be no wage increase during the first six months and 4.5 percent in the second half of the year, part of which (1 percent) would be diverted from the amount scheduled for the training fund for upgrading hospital workers. The arbitrator's award for the second year of the contract was more liberal, a 5 percent increase to go into effect on January 1, 1978. Also there would be larger payments by employers into the benefit funds. The State, after pleading poverty, found $50 to $60 million to advance against future Medicaid and Blue Cross payments. The strike against fifty-seven hospitals and nursing homes finally ended after the workers had been on the streets for eleven days.

In 1978, when the 1199 contract was to expire the Governor called in federal mediators in the face of another strike. The agreement reached gave the union a two-year contract worth 15 percent in wage increases. The governor, the mayor, union and hospital leadership all expressed relief that a strike had been averted.

In 1979 the Committee of Interns and Residents (CIR), a union representing house staff in municipal and voluntary hospitals, called a one-day walkout to protest the quality of care in municipal hospitals. In 1981 CIR staged a seven-day walkout also over quality of care issues in municipal hospitals. The CIR leadership was heavily fined for violation of the New York State Taylor Act and did not win much public or professional support. In essence, the failure of the walkout resulted in the union's becoming a relatively insignificant factor in New York City health politics. With the exception of the CIR activity, the late 1970s to mid–1980s was a period of relative quiescence on the health labor front. There were several reasons for this:

- Governor Carey followed in the footsteps of Governor Rocke-feller in seeking to help unions win wage increases by coming up with State money to avert strikes.
- The precarious state of the New York City and New York State economies, coming out of the fiscal crisis period, exerted a moderating effect on union demands. If any one union won a larger wage increase than any other, the tentative balance might have been upset. There was an effort on the part of union leaders not to unsteady the cart. Thus wage demands were not excessive and not pursued demonstratively.
- The hospital reimbursement system in New York permitted a pass-through of wage increases, meaning that the State would agree to add the new wages to a hospital's reimbursement rate. Under this arrangement the hospitals had no reason to be especially concerned with any wage settlements that were reached.
- The civil service unions in New York City were in a somewhat different position. Wage agreements for these unions (police, fire, government workers, etc.) had to be approved by the Emergency Financial Control Board, set up during the fiscal crisis. This tended to exert a damping effect on the unions' wage demands. This capitulation to the financial recovery of New York City had an impact on nonmunicipal unions as well.

The labor peace was shattered with a forty-seven day strike in the late summer of 1984. The results of the strike were several: the union won a 5 percent wage increase and every other weekend off for its membership (although they could have had 4 percent without a strike); by staying out for so long a time, the union membership lost far more than it gained; and for the first time, the State refused to guarantee money to cover the wage demands and refused to help mediate the strike. In part this was due to the need to keep State health care cost increases below the national average so as not to jeopardize the Medicare waiver and the new hospital reimbursement system.

At the time this book is being written (1985) the implications of this change of events have not become totally evident. What is of interest is the change in leadership of the dominant health workers' union (Local 1199) and the consequences of that change for the union, the health system, and the city.

As noted above, 1199 developed as a largely minority union with a white leadership. While minority members had risen to positions of middle and upper leadership within the union, they did not control the policies of the union. The white leadership had a long history of involvement in progressive causes including the civil rights movement, the anti-war movement and promotion of minority culture and cultural work. Through such activities, the union had won loud acclaim as one of the most democratic of unions and one most concerned with the betterment of its workers. Many of the benefits that 1199 had won involved the ability of workers to receive education aimed at job upgrading and improvement. Nevertheless, many within the rank and file wanted a black president.

With the retirement of Leon Davis in 1982 and the subsequent retirement or death of others in positions of leadership (Moe Foner, Elliot Goodoff, et al.), minority workers began to replace the whites in the union hierarchy. Doris Turner, a black dietician who had worked her way up to vice president was named president and with her came other new officers to succeed the departing whites. While the former leadership had proven skill and long experience in labor negotiations, Turner and her aides did not, having risen to senior positions under the accommodating administrations of Governors Rockefeller and Carey. Thus, the union was headed by new leaders whose ability had never been tested. Other unions, notably District Council 37, will also be experiencing a change in top leadership in the near future; it will be interesting to observe the capability of their successors.

How well did the nonprofessional staff and the nursing staff fare in this twenty-five year period during which several critical developments occurred in the health care arena—the inflow of new dollars, a strong push towards unionization, the increasing numbers of black and Puerto Rican workers in the New York City labor force, the growing importance of public sector trade unions in the politics of the City, and the increasingly powerful role of State government in setting reimbursement rates for hospitals and health care insurance?

The first important finding is that during this period, there was a marked increase in total hospital employment, particularly in the voluntary sector where the numbers almost doubled. A more moderate increase of about one-fifth occurred in the municipal sector. The combined hospital work force increased by about 100,000. In addition, there was a rapid increase in nursing home staffs which reflected the expansion in bed capacity.

The second major development was the significant wage gains that registered nurses and nonprofessional workers achieved. When Local 1199 first organized Montefiore, the annual earnings of low-level workers in voluntary hospitals were in the $1,500 to $1,650 range. The United Hospital Fund's survey of hospital manpower in New York City in 1978 reports the distribution of earnings among key categories of workers in the study's fifty-nine voluntary hospitals (Table 7.3).

After removing the inflationary bias, the lowest paid hospital worker improved his *real* earnings by about threefold over the relatively short period of twenty years—a truly remarkable gain.

But this gain in real income does not tell the whole story. During this period many hospital workers experienced a reduction in their workweek from 44 to 37 hours, roughly a 20 percent decline. Moreover, if they worked overtime they received time and a half pay instead of the straight time or compensating time off that had been the arrangement in 1958.

Another significant change relates to the important gains that hospital workers achieved in their health and welfare benefits. According to our twenty-four hospital analysis, expenditures for this item increased within one decade (1966–1976) by 835 percent in current dollars in comparison with an overall rate of increase of 305 percent.

During these 25 years, workers also achieved additional gains in the form of improved work rules, greater job protection (by limitations on the hospitals' ability to subcontract) and the institution of training opportunities that would provide at least a small minority increased mobility into higher paying classifications.

It would be misreading the evidence to view the entire period as one of uninterrupted gains by workers. A considerable number of hospitals—voluntary, municipal, and proprietary—were closed. Although the State provided special funding to facilitate the hiring of superfluous workers by other medical institutions, only a small number of those who lost their jobs benefited from this program.

There were additional difficulties that the large inflow of money did not resolve. With few exceptions, the municipal hospitals continued to experience shortages of registered nurses which created an adverse working environment for the staff. Nurses had to attend many more

Table 7.3   Earnings for Selected Workers, Voluntary Hospitals, 1978

Housekeeping, property maintenance	$13,000
Administration, general	15,800
Nutrition	12,900
Nursing	15,200

seriously ill patients than they could properly care for, especially at night and on weekends. These arduous shifts, in turn, put the nurses under severe stress.

Moreover, despite the large increases in City tax levy funds and in funds from the State and federal governments, in many municipal hospitals plant and equipment deteriorated and these hospitals found it difficult to acquire new diagnostic and therapeutic equipment.

The municipal hospitals were not the only institutions that faced difficulties in maintaining and improving their levels of operation. The two decades saw the merger and closure of a considerable number of voluntary and proprietary hospitals and a marked deterioration in the capital plant in many leading voluntary hospitals, the full magnitude of which went unnoticed until the major institutions submitted their requests for certificates of need in the early 1980s.

One further challenge concerns the impact of the enlarged dollar inflows on the employment dimensions of the health care system. It is not surprising that the enlarged dollar inflows resulted in a marked expansion in the number of hospital workers and a marked improvement in their wages and working conditions. But, as Victor Gotbaum observed after his last successful negotiation with the City before it entered its fiscal crisis, the gains that his union's members had achieved outstripped those achieved by any other group of comparable workers. What was the concatenation of circumstances that made it possible for hospital workers in both sectors, voluntary and municipal, to achieve gains that were far beyond the gains of other workers in New York City or hospital workers in other areas of the country? Most of the factors that contributed to this unique result have been identified, but in the section that follows, an effort is made to provide a more integrated explanation of the reasons for this accomplishment.

The more than 100 percent increase in the number of hospital employees could not have occurred unless the employing units had been able to improve substantially the wages and working conditions of their employees who in the early post–World War II era had occupied the lowest rungs of the job ladder. The population in New York City had stopped growing; the local economy was strong; more and more opportunities were opening up for young people to remain in the educational system long enough to earn their high school diploma or to go beyond; more opportunities were also available for women. Even poorly educated migrants and immigrants, including many who belonged to minority groups, had alternatives to seeking employment in the hospital sector.

Let us assume that hospitals required many more nursing personnel and nonprofessional workers to provide more care and more intensive levels of care to the patients whom they admitted and treated. Since payroll costs accounted for close to two-thirds of all their costs and since nursing and nonprofessional staff accounted for half of the entire payroll, how could the hospitals cover their vastly increased payrolls? The question needs an answer and a simple answer is found in the improved economic position of hospitals which resulted first from the steadily growing proportion of the population that was covered by hospital insurance and the relative ease with which the public (and particularly the employers who paid for the largest share of this coverage) accepted rapidly rising premiums. This factor played a major role in providing flexibility to the voluntary hospital sector.

As for the municipal hospitals, we find that the local economy was in general strong, there were substantial increases in intergovernmental transfers, and health care and hospitals accounted for no more than about 13 percent of the City's budget. Local revenues provided room for improving the wages and working conditions of all City employees including those employed in its hospitals.

But Blue Cross and commerical insurance and a growing local tax base by themselves would not have enabled the hospitals to respond to the repeated demands of their work force for rising real wages and improved benefits. They key to their response was in the radical change in their revenues that came about after 1965 when Medicare and Medicaid were enacted. For the first time, hospitals were assured of third-party reimbursement, not for a minority but for the vast majority of all patients whom they admitted to their wards and private accommodations. Hospitals could expect retrospective reimbursement which meant that their prior outlays would be covered.

We cannot conclude that this new financial environment for hospitals made them willing to meet the continuing demands of the unions for higher wages and more liberal benefits. However, the hospitals' negotiators did become more forthcoming as they realized that they could receive without too much trouble additional revenues from Blue Cross, commercial insurance, and the federal and state governments to cover the higher wages they had agreed to.

With regard to the City, it initially anticipated that Medicaid would result in a financial bonanza since the federal government would cover half and the State a quarter of the costs for the health and hospital care of the poor. Formerly, the City had been responsible for the entire bill. For a brief time it appeared that the pressure on the City's tax levy would ease while more and more of the costs of public sector health care would be covered through intergovernmental transfers. But this favorable outlook did not last, as the combination of expanded Medicaid rolls, rising health care costs, and the shift of the Medicare beneficiaries out of the municipal hospitals resulted in an increasing, not declining, burden on City tax levy funds. However, until 1974–1975, the City was able to cope, mostly through additional borrowing.

Two more forces played a major role in the story that we are reviewing—the role of unions and the changing political environment in the City and the State. The progress that hospital workers achieved in such a relatively brief period reflected in large measure the strong leadership that Leon Davis provided Local 1199 of the Drug and Hospital Union and Victor Gotbaum's astute direction of District Council 37 of AFSCME. Each had to face difficult intra- and inter-union competition in organizing his union and later in combatting raids. Moreover, while the two could not avoid collision entirely, if they were not to weaken each other, possibly fatally, they had to reach a compromise and they did.

The unions had to make their way initially in an environment in which the law exempted both voluntary and municipal hospitals from having to respond to demands of their workers to enter into collective bargaining. Furthermore, the law prohibited municipal employees from going on strike. To add to these obstacles, growth depended on the union's attracting new members from among black and Puerto Rican groups that had little or no prior experience with unions or with its primarily Jewish leadership.

Supplementing his own considerable strengths, Leon Davis received considerable support from Harry Van Arsdale, the head of the local labor council who was sympathetic to efforts to improve the condition of minority workers, at least in new unions where they were not in direct conflict with the dominant white membership.

On a number of occasions Leon Davis was willing to accept the consequences of defying the law by paying sizable fines and also by spending time in jail, convinced that victory or defeat for his union would finally be determined not by the courts but in the arena of public opinion, a judgment which time corroborated.

Once Mayor Robert Wagner opened the way in 1958–1960 for municipal workers to organize into unions of their own choosing and the City was willing to enter into collective bargaining agreements with these newly formed unions, Victor Gotbaum was quick to appreciate the political leverage that large numbers of well organized City employees provided to him in trading with politicians who sought election or reelection. Such workers would have a major stake in rewarding their friends or punishing their enemies. A mayor who made a good settlement was a friend; one who balked at accepting union demands could not escape the consequences. Organized municipal workers became the most important constituency of every ambitious politician.

For the many years (1959–1973) that Nelson Rockefeller was Governor, the City unions had a good friend in Albany who, it will be remembered, as early as 1963 took the initiative to bring the voluntary hospitals within the scope of the State's labor relations act. And Rockefeller did more. In several critical negotiations in the 1960s and early 1970s, when 1199 and the League of Voluntary Hospitals were deadlocked, the governor let it be known that the hospitals, if they settled, could look to the State for assistance via more liberal reimbursements. This pattern was continued under Governor Carey.

However, even the powerful forces mentioned above would not have enabled the unions to accomplish so much for their members in so short a time unless the citizenry of New York City had been sympathetic and supportive of the demands of the poorly paid hospital workers for improved wages and working conditions. The fact that these workers started so far behind enabled their leadership to repeat the charge of exploitation, even after the facts no longer supported this claim. Small wonder, therefore, that a reaction eventually set in. But even then, hospital workers were still several rungs below workers at, or near, the top of the wage ladder.

8

Assessment

We are now in a position to trace in broad outline the different institutions and groups that were the principal beneficiaries of the large inflow of additional dollars into the health care sector in New York City in the period following the establishment of Medicare and Medicaid in 1966.

To set the stage: between 1966 and 1983, the total dollars flowing into the health care sector increased from approximately $2.5 billion to $16.2 billion or slightly more than sixfold. However, we must eliminate the "inflationary" dimension of this trend if we want to assess what happened to real outputs which were increased by real inputs. To remove the inflationary factor requires that the $2.5 billion base be set at $7.0 billion to adjust for the general inflation that occurred in the consumer price index (CPI) in the New York–New Jersey area during the ensuing period.

At first glance it appears that real inputs increased over the seventeen-year span by over twofold but that conclusion must be modified in two respects. The first modification is that the inflation in medical care costs increased about 15 percent faster than the CPI. That is, the inputs used to provide health care services in 1983 relative to 1966 had risen in price more than the inputs used to produce food, clothing, housing, transportation, and other basic goods. Thus, about $1 billion of the $9.2 billion ($16.2 minus $7.0) that we plan to trace reflects not additional inputs but differentially higher prices.

The other preliminary modification is that the number of people in New York City during the period under study did not remain constant but declined by roughly 10 percent. Therefore, our assessment of what was produced and who the beneficiaries were must take account of this demographic fact: at the end of the period there were slightly over 7 million residents in the City receiving health care services in comparison to about 8 million in the mid–1960s. Although hospitals in New York City have always provided care for a significant minority of nonresidents, we can assume that the proportion of this nonresident population declined during the period under observation as suburban hospitals increased their capacity and their level of sophistication.

There has been a wide-ranging argument among health analysts about the criteria that should be used to assess the value of greater resource use in the provision of health care services. Many analysts contend that the only worthwhile measures of health output are reductions in mortality and morbidity. If more resource inputs lead to additions in the average years of life and concomitant reductions in the amount of illness as reflected in the number of days during which people are bedridden or unable to pursue their normal activities, we have a prima facie case that the additional health care inputs have resulted in useful social output.

But most health analysts balk at such a simplistic approach. To begin with, they point out that improved health care can be reflected not only in the prolongation of human life but in the quality of the patient's remaining years. Modern medical and surgical care have made important contributions to the quality of life for large numbers of persons through hip and knee replacements, the control of hypertension, the care of patients with coronary disease, proven treatment modalities for many neoplastic diseases, effective prostate operations, the removal of cataracts, and many other instances where improved diagnosis and therapy have resulted in greater functionality and less pain.

Even if we were to adopt the criterion of reduced mortality as the best indicator of the value of increased outlays for health care, the last two decades would show significant gains for three critical groups in New York City: the newborn, middle-aged males, and the older elderly.

Infant deaths per 100,000 live births declined in New York City from 4,328 in 1960 to 1,719 in 1980 or from a rate of 26.0 to 16.1 per 1,000 representing a reduction of over 38 percent within the short span of two decades. The rate of decline for New York State and for the United States was even greater: starting at about the same point as the City, their 1980 rates had dropped to 12.5, almost one-quarter below the rate that New York City had been able to achieve.

Much of the explanation for the less satisfactory performance of the City is grounded in several distinctive aspects of its changing demographic profile, the most important of which have been the steep increase in the proportion of the nonwhite population from around 15 percent in 1960 to 40 percent in 1980; the growing proportion of the total population who are living in poverty; and the much higher proportion of out-of-wedlock births which accounted in 1980 for 34.6 of all births in the City, more than double the rate of 17.1 percent for the United States as a whole.

While experts do not agree about the relative contribution of each of the three factors mentioned above to neonatal death rates, they do agree that minority status, low income, and out-of-wedlock births are significant determinants.

There was great restiveness among the nation's health leadership throughout the early post–World War II decades because of the differentially higher death rates among middle-aged American white men; several West European countries showed considerably lower mortality rates for men in the 45 to 65 years age group. Recently, however, the United States experience has become more favorable and the death rates for white men in these pre-retirement years are much improved both in the nation as a whole and in New York City. Finally, during the two decades from 1960 to 1980 during which the City lost about 10 percent of its total population, the number of the older elderly, those above 75, increased from 224,000 to 381,000 or by just under three-fifths.

Even these three indices of reduced infant mortality, sharp reductions in adult white male mortality, and a marked gain in the numbers of the older elderly can be challenged by the extreme positivists who argue that these improvements in health status need not, and should not, be ascribed in the first instance to a larger quantity and better quality of health care services. They ascribe primary credit to improvements in the standard of living and in educational levels, to the reduction in infectious diseases, to the decline in smoking, and to other environmental and behavioral changes.

The importance of environmental factors in assessing health status is underscored by what happened to the homicide rate in New York City and in the United States during the past two decades. As recently as 1960, the rate for both the City and the nation was slightly above 5 per 100,000. By 1970, the City's rate had jumped to 14 and the nation's rate to over 9. In 1980, the City's rate had reached 27 and the national rate stood at 11. When we look at the incidence of homicide by age, sex, and race, we find that it is highest in New York City (and in the nation) among teenage and young adult black males; it is by far the leading cause of death among this subgroup.

In light of the foregoing highly selective review, only a curmudgeon would insist that the additional inflow of real resources into the health care system made no significant contribution to the well-being of the City's population. Nevertheless, it is wrong to assume that all of the increased services, or even most of them, led directly to decreased mortality and morbidity. The truth lies somewhere between.

Since we cannot trace with precision the impact of additional health care services on health care status, the remainder of this assessment will seek to answer in summary fashion two related questions: Who were the principal beneficiaries of the increased services that the system provided? And which provider groups benefited most from the expansion of the health care system?

We will consider a limited number of beneficiary groups. Specifically we will look at the elderly, those over 65 who become eligible for Medicare; those on welfare or close enough to the poverty standard to be eligible for Medicaid; the near-poor who were slightly above the Medicaid standard; the below-65 age group in the middle-income range; the wealthy; the small number of patients who experience major medical problems such as kidney failure requiring renal dialysis; burn victims; and neonates weighing 1,000 grams or less. We will also consider the variability that is introduced into the assessment when consideration is taken of the areas in the City where these groups are concentrated as well as the influence of race on access to health care services.

What were the most noteworthy changes in health care services that became available after 1965 to each of the groups identified above? First, the elderly made considerably greater use of both inpatient and ambulatory care than they had previously. Theirs was the most striking improvement in access to services of all the groups whose experience we are reviewing. Not only did the elderly make considerably greater use of health care services, but they also had access to a better quality of services. The most telling evidence of the latter trend was the shift of large numbers of elderly away from the municipal hospital system which had previously been their major source of inpatient care. After Medicare, they were admitted with greater frequency to voluntary hospitals, including the major teaching hospitals where the quality of care was superior. Many of the elderly, particularly the white elderly who lived in Manhattan and Queens, also had easier access to private practitioners once they became enrolled in Medicare-Part B.

During two critical decades (1960–1980), the nursing home beds in the City were increased about threefold and a higher proportion of the feeble elderly were able to use these facilities. Payment for this kind of care was not covered by government funds except for those who met the Medicaid eligibility standards. However, a considerable number of paying patients, after exhausting their savings, became Medicaid-eligible. In recent years, the City of New York (Department of Human Resources) expanded its program of care for the homebound with an aim of enabling them to remain in their own homes instead of being institutionalized. A high proportion of the 30,000 beneficiaries of this program which cost $400 million in 1983 were the elderly poor who received an average of over fifty hours per week of personal care assistance in their homes paid for by the City.

Many of the elderly whose incomes exceeded the ceiling for Medicaid eligibility were unable to receive any significant government assistance if they sought to cope at home with their increasing disabilities and frailties; they also encountered difficulties if they sought to enter a nursing home. If they found a nursing home able and willing to admit them, they would be responsible for their own bills until all of their assets were exhausted.

Welfare clients and others who were Medicaid-eligible, approximately 1.5 million of the City's 7.1 million population, had expanded access to hospitals, ambulatory care, nursing home care and home care as a result of the legislation in the mid–1960s. While a high proportion continued to seek treatment from neighboring municipal hospitals as they had before the introduction of Medicaid, a significant number sought care elsewhere and were better able to obtain it since the State was willing to reimburse providers. More of the poor received inpatient treatment in voluntary hospitals. But one of the expectations of the new legislation—to bring the poor into the mainstream of American medicine—was not fulfilled because of the decline and, in some areas of the City, the disappearance of private practitioners. The low fees paid to private physicians who treated Medicaid patients also constituted a barrier to these patients' entering the mainstream. Many of the poor had no option but to obtain ambulatory care from a neighboring hospital, community health center, or for-profit Medicaid practice. But these limitations aside, under Medicaid indigent patients saw physicians more frequently than they had in the past.

We have noted previously that many more of the elderly poor were admitted to nursing homes or were certified for home care services and thus avoided premature institutionalization. On balance the poor, as a result of the new dollar inflows, were able to obtain more health care services and those who were hospitalized in major teaching institutions received a higher level of care. But many of the poor, particularly those who lived in the Bronx or the low-income areas of Brooklyn, continued to receive a level of health care far below that obtained by the average citizen.

The experience of the near-poor, some half million people, is the most difficult to assess. Members of this group were not eligible for Medicaid either initially or after the income standards were raised. Many had some hospital insurance but not enough to cover the bills from an extended hospital stay and often their coverage did not include physicians' fees.

While some of the near-poor had used the municipal hospital system for inpatient and even outpatient care, many others had relied on private practitioners and on voluntary hospitals. The acceleration of medical care costs effected by Medicare and Medicaid led to the "monetarization" of the system. This meant that many private physicians who had earlier taken care of patients free or at a reduced charge were no longer willing to do so. In their view, if the patient did not have insurance or could not cover his bill with his own resoures, the responsibility rested with government. Facing the steep rise in per diem costs, voluntary hospitals found that their endowment income was no longer sufficient to cover the free and below-cost care they had previously rendered.

However, several compensatory factors must be taken into account: the breadth and depth of insurance coverage continued to increase; the municipal health care system continued to be available; many community health centers which used a sliding scale of fees became operational; and if an individual with a low income encountered a major medical emergency requiring expensive inpatient treatment, Medicaid would pay. A review of the findings of the 1982 Harris survey for The Commonwealth Fund would not support a conclusion that the near-poor experienced a deterioration in the quantity and quality of health care services over these decades. A more reasonable conclusion is that their access to care did not improve appreciably.

Persons below 65 in the middle-income range, who account for the majority of the City's population, had always had broad access to the comprehensive medical care system that characterized New York City with its large number of practitioners and specialists and its numerous hospitals, voluntary and other, among them some of the most prestigious teaching institutions in the country.

The large dollar flows into the system after the mid–1960s did not affect this large middle-class group. The increasing number of specialists, particularly in Manhattan, reduced the difficulties that many had earlier encountered in getting an appointment with a physician within a few days. But concomitantly the decline in the number of general practitioners made if difficult for many families to find a physician who was willing to assume responsibility for their general medical care. On the other hand, this difficulty should not be exaggerated. Most respondents to the Harris survey reported that they had a regular source of medical care on which they could rely.

Physicians treating middle-class patients who required hospitalization could usually admit them to a hospital immediately, or within a few days, except for the winter months when occupancy, especially in certain leading institutions, was over 90 percent. The closure of a number of proprietary and small community hospitals after 1965 in response to the tightening reimbursement regulations by the State put additional pressure on the voluntary system but not to a point where middle-class patients suffered serious inconvenience. Reductions in average length of stay helped to ease this situation. In addition, the improved quality of insurance coverage enabled many middle-class patients to undergo expensive procedures such as a hip replacement at $15,000 or open heart surgery at $30,000.

Middle-class patients had better access to specialists in private practice and also benefited from the striking advances in the quality of hospital care. The much higher costs of these diagnostic and therapeutic gains did not, however, overburden financially many middle-class patients because their insurance policies increasingly covered "major medical expenses." Only a very few patients encountered a catastrophic illness that invaded much or all of their savings.

Since the vast majority of middle-income persons below the age of 65 had improved access after 1965 to ambulatory and hospital care, it follows that the affluent minority, those in the upper income brackets, were in an even better position. This minority had always had access to the full range of health care services—preventive and rehabilitative as well as therapeutic. But in the post–1965 period, the insurance coverage of members of this upper income group began to include extended outpatient psychiatric treatment, annual physical examinations, physical therapy and other rehabilitative services. Many of the affluent had access to these services without having to pay for them directly.

One last group consists of patients in need of very expensive medical treatment. The outstanding example is a patient requiring renal dialysis. The 1972 amendments to the Social Security Act made the federal government responsible for covering 80 percent of the costs of their treatment, which currently comes to over $30,000 a year per patient.

Third-party payment which covers over 90 percent of all hospital expenditures encouraged a number of large medical centers to establish treatment facilities for burn victims or for low birth weight neonates. The hospital bill for the more expensive episodes often exceeds $100,000. The large inflow of new funds into the system made it possible for selected institutions to pioneer in treating various categories of high risk patients, often with great success.

We have seen that the new large dollar inflows had the following results:

- The Medicaid population had easier access to more and better inpatient, nursing home, and home care services.

- The near-poor had to seek more of their care from public medical institutions.
- The middle and upper income groups had access to more and better ambulatory and inpatient care with reduced out-of-pocket payments.
- Selected groups of patients requiring expensive episodic or continuing treatment were able to obtain it at little or no cost.

To round out this recital, note should be taken of the questionable results of the policy of early discharge of hospitalized mental patients. New York State, like many other states, decided to speed the release of chronic mental patients to their own communities where they could be treated on an outpatient basis. The accelerated efforts at deinstitutionalization were surely encouraged by the budgetary benefits that they conferred upon the State. Most of the costs of maintenance and medical care for these patients were transferred to the federal government. Maintenance costs were largely covered by the Supplemental Security Income program (SSI). Medical costs for the elderly became the responsibility of Medicare, of Medicaid for the younger patients. In addition a large number of senile patients were simply transferred to a nursing home, which was reimbursed by Medicaid.

However, many deinstitutionalized patients cannot get along without the support of a structured hospital environment; they are unable to make or maintain contact with psychiatric resources in their community; they cannot find suitable housing; and they are subject to exploitation by unscrupulous persons. Deinstitutionalization has proved not to be a panacea for all the mentally ill.

We are now ready to consider the question of how the additional dollars that flowed into the health care system were distributed among the different providers. To put this issue in perspective, we should recall that we must account for over an additional $9 billion which were available for distribution in 1983 in comparison with 1966.

There are two approaches we can pursue in tracing these enlarged outlays for health care. The first is to focus on the principal institutional providers to learn how they fared during this expansionary period. The second is to look more closely at specific groups of personnel in and outside these institutions and assess their gains.

On the institutional front, we know that the proprietary hospitals in New York failed to benefit from the large increase in dollar flows and between 1960 and 1980 many closed. In 1981 only 7.3 percent of all general care beds were still in proprietary hospitals, down from 11.8 percent in 1958. These facilities have never achieved more than a marginal place in the City's hospital structure.

The second clear-cut finding is that the large municipal hospital system was not strengthened by the substantial addition of new funds flowing into health care, although most of these funds stemmed from enlarged federal and State outlays. The number of municipal hospitals shrank from twenty-one in 1958 to twelve in 1981 and the proportion of inpatient days in these hospitals declined from 21.7 to 17.5 percent of the total during the same period. While the municipal system demonstrated more resiliency in the arena of ambulatory care, even here it lost part of its share (several percentage points) to voluntary hospitals.

In assessing the voluntary hospital sector, small community hospitals must be differentiated from large hospitals with graduate training programs and from the major medical centers. Several small voluntary hospitals closed and several others were merged. We can tentatively infer from this that small institutions found it difficult to stay afloat as medicine became more sophisticated and residents became critical for the provision of inpatient care.

The prospects for community hospitals to survive and prosper depended greatly on their location. When most of the middle-class clientele that were the mainstay of their staff's practices moved out of the area and were replaced by minority and low-income groups, inner-city hospitals faced major difficulties in remaining fiscally viable. A number of community hospitals in Brooklyn, the Bronx and even in Manhattan had to close or merge. In the case of Polyclinic-French Hospital (over 400 beds) located in mid-Manhattan, bankruptcy was compounded by the bad judgment of its trustees who purchased the New Yorker Hotel and found after they had done so that it could not be easily converted into a hospital facility.

Even major teaching hospitals which serve as the primary affiliates of a medical school defy simple generalizations. One, Flower Fifth Avenue,' was converted into a nursing home in the late 1970s after New York Medical College moved to Westchester County. New York University was able to build a University Hospital which was opened in 1963. At the beginning of the 1980s, Presbyterian, Mt. Sinai, and New York Hospital were using substantially the same facilities that had been in place in the 1930s except for some specialized new construction linked to their expanding research activities.

The 400-bed University Hospital at Einstein Medical College tried to operate as an independent institution, not once but twice, but concluded that it could survive only if it became integrated with the much larger Montefiore Hospital and Medical Center. For the Downstate University Hospital in Brooklyn, no similar merger opportunities were available although a 1983 special consultants' report

recommended that the president of Downstate explore various alternatives including closer linkages with several other teaching hospitals
affiliated with Downstate Medical School.

Major construction proposals were submitted by New York Hospital, Mt. Sinai, and Presbyterian to the State of New York for approval
in 1982. These proposals precipitated the appointment of the Hyman
Committee and a State-wide moratorium on certificate of need ap-
provals. These large construction requests, primarily for renovation
and modernization, each in the $400 million range, called attention to
the poor state of the capital plant of each of the hospitals, much of it
dating back to the 1920s or even earlier. Although many new dollars
flowed into the hospital system after 1965, the tight controls exercised
by the State over reimbursement did not permit these institutions to
accumulate sufficient surplus to finance large-scale capital projects.
The trustees and administrators, responding to physicians' pressures,
acted favorably with respect to purchases of new equipment and the
establishment of new services while they neglected the upkeep and
modernization of their plants. By 1982 the long-term neglect had
caught up with each of these institutions and could no longer be
ignored.

Despite the large flow of new dollars into the system over the better
part of two decades, in 1984 most of the major hospitals in New York
City were in less than optimal positions, primarily because of short-
falls in capital investment. This is the case not only with respect to the
prestigious medical centers we have just identified but also of other
large teaching hospitals such as St. Luke's–Roosevelt as well as several
of the major municipal hospitals including Kings County, Bronx
Municipal Hospital Center, and Queens. Although there have been
some notable gains in new construction at Lenox Hill, Memorial, St.
Vincent's, and others, overall the hospital plant in the City has deteriorated in the last two decades.

Reference should also be made to the addition of a number of
freestanding and satellite ambulatory care centers that were established during the last two decades, many of them prior to 1972, which
provide medical care to low-income families living in areas of the City
which have suffered an erosion in the number of general practitioners. A United Hospital Fund estimate suggests that these centers
may provide up to one-quarter of all ambulatory care visits provided
by hospital clinics and emergency rooms in the City.

New sources of public financing undergirded the expansion of
these clinics in at least two ways. The federal government, with occa-
sional contributions from State government, helped these clinics get
started, and the availability of Medicare, Medicaid, and other govern-

ment reimbursement for eligible categories of patients provided the principal share of their operating funds.

The final institutional provider that should be included in this assessment is the nursing home, for-profit and nonprofit. Together, these nursing homes expanded their bed capacity during the two decades by about threefold. The fact that Medicaid provided reimbursement for patients in nursing homes who met its eligibility standards, either prior or subsequent to admission after they had exhausted their own resources, was a direct spur to the expansion of nursing home beds. Public dollars came to account for more than half of all revenues. It is likely that in the absence of Medicaid, the nursing home capacity in the City might have increased slightly to accommodate a larger number of the elderly infirm who could afford to pay their own way or have their way paid by their children or other relatives; but without government financial support, the expansion would have been much more modest.

The revenues received by health care institutions—academic medical centers, hospitals, clinics, nursing homes—are paid in turn to different groups who are directly engaged in producing the services or who help to maintain the institution in which the services are provided. The other part of the funds which the institution receives go to cover the nonpersonnel costs which include new equipment, consumables such as fuel, food and medical supplies, various forms of insurance, and still other essentials. In the early 1960s, payroll costs plus fringe benefits approximated two-thirds of all hospital outlays; by the end of the next decade their share had dropped some 10 percentage points, but payroll still represented more than half of all expenditures.

In tracing the flow of dollars to various groups of employees, we will consider in turn physicians, nurses and allied health personnel, housekeeping, dietary, clerical, and senior administrative personnel.

The substantial inflow of new monies for reimbursement of hospital-based physicians under both Medicare A and B as well as under Medicaid, together with increased sums flowing in via Blue Cross/ Blue Shield and commercial insurance, enabled the major medical centers and their principal affiliated hospitals to increase substantially the number of residents and supervisory physicians and concomitantly to provide them with improved stipends and salaries for their part- or full-time work schedules. While the stipends for residents almost tripled over the two decades, an increase that was in line with inflation, that does not tell the whole story. Because of the vastly enlarged sums flowing into all facets of the medical care system, a resident willing to work hard—36 hours over a weekend—can currently earn as much as $1,000. And a considerable number, especially in the later years of their residency, avail themselves of such opportunities.

The large medical centers and their principal teaching affiliates would not have been able to attract and retain this many senior supervisory physicians without the new sources of funds that became available via the reimbursement route. In many specialties, these major hospital centers were able to offer for the first time in the history of fee-for-service medicine a package of salary, fringe benefits, work schedule, vacation and other benefits for senior clinicians that was reasonably competitive with what these physicians could earn in private practice. Not infrequently, the arrangements enabled those on salaries to engage in stipulated amounts of private practice that would further enhance their total earnings.

As is often the case, however, the new favorable arrangements that became available for the full-time staff (or geographic full-time staff) had adverse consequences for other physicians, especially attending physicians who had volunteered their services for treating the poor and participating in educational programs. In most major academic health centers the voluntary staff were seen as an anachronism; their services were no longer sought after or valued. When some clinical departments introduced physician practice plans which required a pooling of earnings, part of it to be earmarked for the institution and part for the department, many of the long-term voluntary staff resigned. We are still a long way from the dualism that characterizes medical care in Great Britain or in Germany where a sharp differentiation exists between the hospital staff and practitioners in the community, but we have surely moved in that direction in the large teaching hospitals in New York City and in other major urban centers. The odds are that this movement will continue.

Despite the steeply rising costs of practice from malpractice premiums, rent, and office personnel, the number of specialists engaged in private practice in Manhattan continued to increase even in the face of a declining patient population. The best explanation for this counter-intuitive trend is the larger amount of money available for patients to spend for specialty care and the longer hours that the specialists had to treat paying patients. Physicians were able to maintain and improve their incomes by cutting back or eliminating the time that they used to donate to the poor. Moreover, Medicare and other third parties, except for Medicaid, were willing to meet their steadily rising fees.

General practitioners and other primary care physicians who practiced in middle-class neighborhoods fared less well. The younger

among them tended to follow their patients as they relocated to the
suburbs and the older group retired earlier than they had planned.
From the middle 1970s on, even the well-trained young diplomate
found it increasingly difficult to become established as a specialist,
unless he or she were taken on as a junior partner by a senior
physician.

Underservice of the outer boroughs and even of sections of Manhattan offered opportunities for many FMGs, including US-FMGs, to
obtain a place on the periphery if not in the center of private, hospital,
or clinic practice. They had to work hard for their money, often in
unattractive treatment settings, but these shortcomings aside, the con-
fluence of Medicare and Medicaid funding together with the declining presence of U.S. medical school graduates enabled many of these
newly trained and licensed FMGs to establish a practice; by the mid–
1970s they accounted for about half of all practitioners in New York
City.

Two concluding observations: a single average of physicians' incomes in New York City in the early 1980s compared to the mid–1960s
would obscure almost as much as it would reveal. Dispersions around
the mean are substantial. There is reason to believe from the scattered
information that is available that established specialists have done well
over these two decades even after taking into consideration the inflation and the increasing costs of practice.

An economist must note that in the face of the rising number of
physicians per 100,000, one would have anticipated a marked decline
in the earnings of most physicians. No one contends that such a
decline occurred although there is disagreement about the magnitude
of the gains in real income. The flow of new funds into the health care
system surely underpinned the increasing real incomes of most physicians in New York City.

The impact of the increased dollar flows on nursing personnel and
on allied health professionals is even more complex to summarize. In
nursing, we must distinguish among a small number of senior nurses
in administrative positions, the much larger number of registered
nurses, the substantial numbers of licensed practical nurses, and the
many who are grouped under the classification "nurses' aides."

The first impact of the additional dollars was to strengthen the
demand for all types of nursing personnel; the total numbers employed in hospitals and nursing homes more than doubled. Nevertheless, several times during the two decades, a number of general care
hospitals found it difficult to recruit and retain their targeted number
of registered nurses. The municipal hospitals faced a continuing
shortfall in registered nurses resulting from a combination of lagging

salary adjustments (compared to the voluntary hospitals), the reluc-
tance of nurses to travel into unsafe neighborhoods, and the inadequate staffing in many municipal hospitals which added to an already
arduous assignment. Looking at the beginning and the end of the
period, it is hard to find striking gains in the real income of registered
nurses although their fringe benefits and working conditions improved.

Licensed practical nurses, particularly those on the payrolls of the
municipal hospitals, have probably been the greatest beneficiaries of
the increased funds flowing into the health care system. They represent the backbone of the nursing service not only in municipal hospitals but also in nursing homes and to a lesser extent in home health
care. In 1982 the licensed practical nurse earned about 80 percent of
the basic salary of the registered nurse.

Over the two decades, there has been a major increase in the
salaries of the top echelon of the nursing services in both the large
voluntary and the municipal hospitals in growing recognition of the
contribution that senior nurse administrators can make to efficiency.
The salary schedule for other nurses remains compressed with charge
and head nurses and clinical specialists earning only slightly more
than general duty nurses.

The thrust of the foregoing has been to highlight that the primary
impact of the additional dollars on nursing was to broaden substantially the numbers who were employed. However, the fact that so
many additional nurses were available for employment acted as a
constraint on the rise in their real earnings.

It is impossible to generalize about the economic progress of the
large and differentiated numbers of allied health professionals and
nonprofessionals. A few categories such as radiology technicians did
well—that is, their earnings increased more than those of the average
technician. But for the most part, the increases in wages of these
workers lagged behind those of both physicians and the unskilled.

As we saw in the last chapter, nonprofessional personnel at both
voluntary and municipal hospitals experienced sizable gains in both
salaries and fringe benefits during the decades under review. Their
earnings increased more than two-and-one-half fold within the two
decades, their work schedules were reduced, and they received many
valuable fringe benefits.

The final group is the middle and senior hospital administrators.
Their numbers, salaries, and perquisites increased substantially. Several factors contributed to their increase: first, the professionalization
of their work as reflected in the additional education and training
which they acquired before and while they were on the job; next, an
increase in the complexity of their work as a result of the combined

influences of a larger inflow of dollars and a more tightly regulated environment within which they had to operate; competition for managerial talent inside and outside of the health care arena which made hospital trustees willing to restructure the administrative salary scale; finally, the fact that top administrators of the large hospitals, like senior executives of major corporations, were in a strategic position to take good care of themselves and their deputies.

This then is what the enlarged inflow of dollars brought to different groups of patients and providers:

- The number and quality of health care services—inpatient, ambulatory, and nursing home—increased substantially. The principal beneficiaries were the elderly, the poor, and certain patients requiring expensive treatments. The rest of the population obtained access to more sophisticated care.
- The institutional beneficiaries were the strong academic health centers and their large teaching affiliates. The proprietary system and the municipal system declined, absolutely and relatively, as did many small voluntary hospitals. The nursing home sector underwent a substantial expansion.
- Among those engaged in providing health care services, physicians as a whole did well. Impressive gains were made by salaried staff at the major teaching hospitals and established specialists in private practice. Among the nonphysician groups, the top rungs of the nursing profession and hospital administration did well. Licensed practical nurses and nonprofessional hospital personnel also experienced marked improvements in earnings and working conditions.

This assessment points up that selected groups of physicians, who were well entrenched when the money inflows accelerated, were able to maintain and improve their position and that selected nonphysician providers, through a combination of market forces and trade union and political activity, were also able to make significant gains. Among institutions, the large teaching hospitals improved their positions but despite the new sums entering the system, they could not avoid the deterioration of their physical plants.

9

Lessons for the Future

The future is certain to be different from the past. In an arena such as health care, where knowledge and technology are characterized by rapid improvement and the existing financial base cannot remain constant, the future is likely to be substantially different. Nevertheless, a broad assessment of the impact of the increased dollar inflows upon the structure and functioning of the health care system in New York City should provide lessons with applicability for the future. This chapter will extract a few of these lessons.

Lesson number one is that money flowing into the health care system which is aimed at improving access to medical care for designated groups of patients, such as the elderly and the poor, can accomplish at least part of its specific goal. In New York City, as in the nation as a whole, Medicare, Medicaid, and special federal and State funding for health services enabled both the elderly and the poor to obtain more and better health care. Although it has become intellectually fashionable to argue that government is unable to set and accomplish useful social objectives and that throwing money at problems, as the phrase goes, seldom accomplishes a worthwhile goal, a review of the last two decades of the health care delivery system in New York City defies this negative conclusion.

What is true, and this is lesson number two, is that the infusion of large amounts of new money, especially from the public sector, is likely to lead to consequences that were not considered in the planning phase. Furthermore, some of the consequences that are anticipated will not occur. Let us consider each of these outcomes in turn.

During the several years when the proposal of Medicare was being actively debated, neither its proponents nor opponents considered the inflationary effect it was likely to have on the whole of the health care sector and particularly on hospital care. To obtain a grudging acceptance of Medicare by the American Medical Association, President Johnson agreed that the federal government would avoid interfering with existing physician/patient relations which were predicated on fee-for-service payment. This conciliatory gesture contributed to the escalation of costs which followed, but in any case, the acceleration would have been more rapid than most experts anticipated because no one could foresee the full consequences of an increase in the proportion of third-party reimbursements for hospital care from 30 to 40 percent of the total to 80 or 90 percent.

The other theme imbedded in this lesson relates to the anticipated results which did not eventuate. Many knowledgeable persons on both sides of the issue about the proper role for the federal government in paying for health care for the poor and the elderly anticipated that if the legislation were passed providers would be swamped. It was believed that physicians and hospitals would be unable to cope with the pent-up demand. But in New York City and in most other urban areas, demand did not outpace supply beyond creating a temporary imbalance. The demand for medical care did increase but not at a runaway rate and the system demonstrated considerable adaptability. Hospitals in particular were flexible; they were able to admit and treat more patients by reducing their average length of stay and by adding to their professional and support personnel.

Lesson number three relates to the dangers that threaten when proponents of new policies set overly ambitious goals. There was considerable discussion before and after the legislation was passed to the effect that it was important for the public sector to assume a larger role in the financing of health care so that all persons, the elderly and the poor as well as the rest of the society, would be included within mainstream medicine. The proponents of an increased role for the federal government argued that the United States needed and that all of its citizens were entitled to the same high level of health care which the middle and the upper classes enjoyed.

It is not necessary to challenge the underlying principle that in matters of relief of pain, recovery of function, and above all the enjoyment of life, a person's capital and income should not determine his or her access to therapeutic and rehabilitative services but that all citizens by virtue of their humanity and membership in the polity should have broadly equal access to the services of health care providers. But if this principle is ethically sound, it does not follow that without modification it can inform public policy. If its pursuit holds little promise of being realized in fact, its propagation can only contribute to later frustration when the test of reality finds it lacking.

More than other cities, New York City had made special efforts to provide reasonable access to health care for its less favored groups but no one acquainted with the history of its municipal health care system would presume that even a large inflow of new public dollars would enable racial minorities, the foreign speaking, the uneducated, the poor, and the frail elderly with no independent means to obtain access to the range and quality of health care services that were available to the businessman, the professor, the civil servant, the electrician, and others who had savings and disposable income which permitted wide-ranging choices.

Though exaggerated, the expectation of a single level of health care for all was, nevertheless, partially fulfilled. The elderly and even a significant proportion of the poor were admitted for inpatient treatment to the best voluntary hospitals in the City. Moreover, Park Avenue specialists were pleased to accept Medicare patients especially if they were able to make up the difference between the physicians' charges and the maximum fee allowed by the federal government.

On the other hand, the Medicaid population was never welcomed by the City's more successful practitioners and specialists. Aside from the low reimbursement fees allowed by the State for office visits, the presence of large numbers of Medicaid patients in waiting rooms was deemed to be unattractive by physicians who catered to middle and upper class patients with the means to pay their way or with private insurance coverage.

Nowhere was the distinction by level of service sharper than in the nursing homes. While a number of Medicaid patients who obtained admission to nursing homes subsidized by philanthropic funds received adequate care, the majority had to accept a marginal level of care that characterized the proprietary nursing homes available to persons with limited or no private means.

The lesson that emerges from this attenuated discussion is that the newly available funds might have gone further and provided better services for the poor, had we recognized at the outset the potential benefit of channelling these dollars to selected groups of hospitals, clinics, and private providers committed to meeting certain explicit standards rather than casting the additional revenues into a highly fragmented market. Belatedly, the mayor and the governor have begun to design some modest experiments to determine whether linking Medicaid patients to a limited number of providers can improve services and control costs.

Related to but distinguishable from the foregoing lesson is the danger of political action without prior discussion. Medicaid was appended to Medicare at the last moment, largely through the persuasive power of Wilbur Cohen, then Under-Secretary of HEW, in his negotiations on behalf of the Johnson Administration with Wilbur Mills, the Chairman of the Ways and Means Committee of the House of Representatives. Since from the start Medicaid was a federal-state, and in a few states such as New York a federal-state-local, program, it could have benefited from the inputs of governors and mayors. But the exigencies of the legislative process did not permit such consultation. The president, with a strong assist from Cohen, recognized it was then or an indefinite delay, and the president came down in favor of then.

The lack of understanding of the impact of the new legislation on state and local governments is nowhere better illustrated than in the case of New York State and New York City. Governor Rockefeller's enabling legislation made one-third of the State's population Medicaid-eligible and Mayor Lindsay and his staff, impressed by the 75 percent combined reimbursement rate from the federal and state governments, believed that the new legislation was a financial bonanza which held promise of helping to solve the City's increasingly strained finances. This led the City and State to undertake a major recruiting drive for eligibles. But within the short span of two years both the governor and the mayor realized that they had miscalculated and were forced to adopt a constrictive rather than an expansionary policy which has bedeviled the program from that day to this, particularly after the State set a low reimbursement rate for visits to physicians and later, in the mid-1970s, began to prune the lists of eligibles.

A policy which expanded and then reduced the flow of public funding together with a policy which built up the roll of eligibles and then pared it down played havoc with the expectations of the citizenry and also created operating difficulties for providers who expanded their operation to cope with the added work load and then found that the funding had been radically reduced.

Lesson number five, foreshadowed by the foregoing, states that every level of government—federal, state, and local—will have to adopt a more cautious stance when a service commands a significant part of its total budget. When Medicare and Medicaid were first placed on the statute books, the federal government's total outlays for health care were quite small, both in absolute terms, $5 billion, and relative to the rest of its budget, which in 1966 amounted to $118.4 billion. Most state governments including the State of New York had outlays for health care that were limited to the support of mental patients and a few others who required institutional care plus some responsibility for general hospital care for low-income persons and the elderly. By the early 1970s, the steep acceleration in health care costs had begun to have an adverse impact on the budgets of all three levels of government and since then the pressures have become more acute. In the federal budget, health care costs have been, and continue to be, the most steeply rising outlays. And both New York State and New York City have been under increasing budgetary pressures because of the need to spend more and more for health.

The lesson that emerges from this abbreviated discussion is that once the outlay for a specific service comes to command a significant and growing proportion of a government's budget, it is inevitable that the legislators will reconsider their previously expansionary stance and attempt to dampen future outlays. The necessity of raising additional revenues led legislators to moderate their enthusiasm for even popular programs such as the expansion of health services.

Most governmentally financed programs are controlled by defining the numbers of eligible persons and by setting an annual budgetary cap on the total outlays. In Medicare and Medicaid, however, both the federal and some state governments relaxed their practice of tightly defining the eligible group and further committed themselves to cost reimbursement rather than a budgetary approach. The federal government alone is in a position to spend money in excess of the amounts that it is able to raise via taxes and even the federal government cannot pursue deficit financing indefinitely without causing a series of dysfunctional effects such as accelerating inflation, raising interest rates to excessively high levels, or starting and stopping the economy in a way that produces excessive unemployment and retards growth.

When Medicare and Medicaid were added to the statute books of the federal and state governments, little prior consideration had been given to the methods whereby providers, particularly hospitals, were to be reimbursed. Blue Cross and commercial insurance and a limited number of governmentally financed health programs had reimbursed hospitals on a retrospective basis and this pattern was adopted in the case of Medicare and Medicaid. When third-party payers accounted for between 80 and 90 percent of all hospital expenditures, it soon became clear that few restraints remained to encourage trustees and hospital administrators to exercise caution in their outlays. In the past, these hospital leaders had been careful to spend no more than they received from the patients they treated plus funds available from endowment or through philanthropic efforts. But once third parties covered the expenditures of eight or nine out of every ten patients and did so in terms of the hospitals' posted charges or audited costs, the basic equation of dollars out to dollars in was fundamentally altered. Hospitals suddenly were in an environment in which the more they spent, the better. There was no point to their continuing to pursue fiscally conservative policies. In fact, they ran the risk of losing out to competitors unless they acquired the most recent equipment, often before its efficacy had been fully established; unless they added more professional and support staff to increase the flow of patients they could treat; unless they raised salaries and fringe benefits and thus attracted and retained better professional and support staffs.

Within a few years of the establishment of Medicare and Medicaid the State of New York as well as a number of other states found it necessary to constrain the accelerating increases in the premium rates for Blue Cross and to slow their outlays for Medicaid by moving first moderately, and later vigorously, to a system of prospective reimbursement.

It must be admitted that government regulation of prices which has been the established method for the sale of electric power, railroads, urban transportation, the telephone company, and several other basic services has brought problems. But this "public utility" approach faced additional difficulties when applied to the hospital sector with its large number of different hospitals providing a range of different services, to different populations, in different locations.

Despite these difficulties, most states that opted for regulation have continued to rely on it, convinced that the total costs to government, insurance, and the public are several percentage points below those of states that have continued to use a charge or cost-reimbursement approach. Prospective reimbursement is currently receiving a nation-wide test based on the federal government's instituting the diagnosis-related group (DRG) system of reimbursing hospitals for the care of Medicare patients. The DRGs represent a radical innovation in reimbursement policy; the more surprising fact, however, is that it has taken the federal government eighteen years to explore an alternative to cost reimbursement.

The lesson that emerges here is that when any group of providers is freed from the constraints of the marketplace and their expenditures are not predetermined by government allocations and/or by the sums that they are able to raise from philanthropic contributions they no longer have to face the test of the *marginal* economic and social value of their output. If churches, schools, social welfare agencies, even police departments were able to spend whatever they considered reasonable on the assumption that these expenditures would add to the well-being of individuals and the community, we would have a close analogue to the conditions under which most hospitals have operated during the last two decades. But this freedom cannot be granted to any group in the society if the society must balance expenditures among competing valuable and desired services.

This last discussion brings us to lesson number seven which New York City's experience addresses directly. A civilized society cannot deny basic health services to individuals and groups who are unable to pay for them. Since antiquity, religious orders have assumed an obli-

gation to assist the sick and injured. Even when medicine had relatively little to offer by way of cure, palliation, comfort, and spiritual
support were provided by those who were committed to pursuing
good works.

Through its elaborate public health care program which included
clinics, visits by nurses to the patients at home, hospitals, long-term
care facilities, and payments to physicians on behalf of welfare patients, the City of New York has demonstrated its commitment to
providing essential health care services to the poor and the indigent.
But for many decades prior to 1965 the City did not preempt the
arena but pursued policies that encouraged the voluntary sector to do
as much as possible to help the poor obtain essential medical care.
Moreover, through budgetary allocations, the City exercised tight
control over the proportion of its total outlays devoted to this important social purpose which ranked only behind fire and police, education, and public assistance in order of importance.

Health care financing in the United States depends on government
for about two-fifths, on insurance for over one-quarter, and for the
remainder, less than one-third, on out-of-pocket payments by the
consumer. In New York City the government's share is considerably
higher, about 60 percent. There is no effective model in this or any
other country of fitting these three sources of payment together into a
framework that will assure access for all who need care and at the
same time not lead to excessive total expenditures.

The burden of lesson seven, then, is that the long-time pattern of
government's responsibility for the health care of the poor which had
worked with reasonable success in New York City was jettisoned when
the new entitlement programs were established. It was assumed that
the enlarged flow of government dollars would assure the poor more
and better services. And, as we noted in lesson number one, the new
government dollars achieved a part of this objective. As long as
physicians in private practice and voluntary hospitals continue to be
the dominant providers of medical care, it is problematic whether
government dollars alone will assure the poor broad access to the
system. The poor must remain a shared responsibility of both the
public and private sectors.

Lesson number eight notes that in a dynamic sector such as health
care, in a dynamic economy and society such as the United States,
even large-scale government initiatives such as the health legislation of
1965 can address only the issues of the day. Sooner or later, new
problems will inevitably arise and demand attention and new solu-
tions must be developed to respond to them.

Many of the health care reformers who played key roles in cultivat-
ing the climate for the passage of Medicare and Medicaid looked

upon the new programs as an interim move that would propel the health care system one step closer to national health insurance which they believed would provide the long-term answer. In their view, the next step in the process would be the passage by Congress of an entitlement program covering all mothers and children and when that had been accomplished they expected the momentum to bring all other uninsured adults within the federal program, the last step in this long campaign.

The legislative proposal to provide coverage for all mothers and children did not go very far because of the mounting financial pressures exerted by rising Medicare and Medicaid outlays which led even liberally inclined congressmen to adopt a wait-and-see approach. Moreover, the proponents of the proposal to expand health insurance with federal dollars could not demonstrate the need for a national entitlement program since Medicaid covered poor mothers and children and improved insurance was available for the middle class.

All three levels of government—the federal government, New York State, and New York City—moved to reduce, not increase, health care outlays by putting in place control programs including utilization reviews, areal planning, certificates of need for capital outlays, reductions in hospital beds and in duplicated services, and still other approaches. The lesson that becomes clear is that any significant departure such as Medicare and Medicaid which turns out to have long-term unanticipated financial consequences for public budgets will force the affected levels of government to intervene with untried and untested policies and programs to staunch the outflow of public funds.

Lesson number nine helps to flesh out this abstract formulation of the ratchet effect between a large-scale governmental initiative and the subsequent interventions aimed at assisting payers to correct course. As indicated earlier, New York State took increasingly strong actions to moderate the rise in health and hospital reimbursements and insurance premiums in the 1970s. One concomitant effect of this State effort was to reduce the operating margins of hospitals. For some years in the mid–1970s several of the major academic health centers in New York City had to draw down their endowments to cover their operating expenses. They were in no position to build up equity to cover future construction needs.

This adaptation led to unexpected and undesirable consequences. In the early 1980s the State recognized for the first time that the major medical institutions in New York City would no longer defer maintenance and avoid rebuilding their aging plants. Their combined requests for certificates of need were in the $2 billion range. Caught off balance, the State resorted to a one-year moratorium (1983), but at its expiration it had to lift the moratorium and grant selected approvals with the plans somewhat scaled down and the proposals somewhat more responsive to areal as well as institutional needs.

This dilemma that confronts New York State is not an aberration; just the opposite. Politicians always choose to avoid current pain since they may no longer be in office and may not have to take responsibility for untoward circumstances in the future. Consider the deteriorating infrastructure at every level of government—the national highway system, New York State's prisons, many of New York City's hospitals, schools, parks, bridges, subways. And neglect is not exclusively a public sector shortcoming. Many critics contend that the decreasing competitiveness of U.S. industry is directly linked to decisions by chief executive officers to underinvest in order to improve their balance sheets.

Distressed by the accelerating expenditures for health care induced and stimulated by Medicare and Medicaid, a number of economists and politicians have recently advanced the theory that the only way out of the current difficulties is to re-establish the competitive market as the key mechanism for determining how much of the nation's resources should be directed to health care. Since we have identified some of the difficulties flowing from a policy of regulating the health care sector, an alternative approach that would diminish or eliminate the role of government would be attractive. However, if the large increase in federal and state dollars did not accomplish what had been expected of it, other simplistic nostrums such as a shift from government regulation to reliance on the competitive market should be carefully scrutinized.

Several points: the competitive market has never been firmly established in the health care sector, therefore we cannot talk of re-establishing it. History will not provide much guidance. Since government funds currently account for over two-fifths of all expenditures for health care, we cannot set up the competitive market as the arbiter. If the access of the poor and the near-poor to the health care system continues to be a social imperative, the continuing responsibility and role of government cannot be eliminated.

Let us grant that the last decades of greater government regulation in many states, including New York, present an equivocal record in which it is difficult to determine the balance between gains and losses. We know that the market has worked well in some sectors of the economy but not in others. And we have no experience with which to foretell how it will perform in health care. An important lesson from the last two decades is that the American people must adopt a skeptical stance toward any simplistic solution. We have paid a substantial price to learn that dollars alone cannot achieve priority health goals.

Therefore, we must be alert to guard against a new theory that promises both to do more and at the same time to save dollars.

The tenth and final lesson is that the health care system is the product of history in which the following powerful forces have played and continue to play a major role:

- Physicians who, after a lengthy period of training, are licensed by the state to exercise broad decision-making powers in the diagnosis and treatment of patients who seek their advice and counsel
- Voluntary hospitals, much of whose capital has been contributed by local philanthropy, which continue to attract to their boards a significant number of the community's leaders
- Insurance carriers which, since World War II, have succeeded in providing coverage for most expensive hospital care and a high proportion of physician's services
- A large and diversified work force consisting of professionals other than physicians, allied health personnel, and large numbers of relatively unskilled workers who depend for their jobs, their income and their status on the continuing vitality of the health care sector
- The educational-research establishment which carries primary responsibility for the basic and advanced training of all physicians and most other health professionals, their contributions to new knowledge and technique being the key factors in the ongoing transformation of the system
- Government which has a great many different responsibilities including the direct financing of the medical care of a significant proportion, about one in four, of the total population.

Each of the foregoing has a distinct relationship to the health care system with distinct goals, commitments, and power to influence how the system changes, in what directions, and at what speed. But that means that no one sector, not even the federal government, can by itself reshape the system.

The characteristic pluralism of the U.S. health care system must be accepted as a basic fact in all discussions affecting its reform and reconstruction. A second basic fact is the difference in views and outlook of the multiple groups that are involved in the ongoing operation of the system. The final fact is that under the impetus of new knowledge and new technology the extant system is constantly undergoing changes, many of which are likely to have far reaching effects.

If we accept, as we must, these critical dimensions as fundamental characteristics of our health care system, then certain policy implications inevitably follow. The first and most important is that there is no single new departure that, by itself, will resolve most of the current problems that demand attention. This means that our concern about cost inflation which has been at the top of the nation's health agenda for more than a decade is unlikely to be resolved through the introduction of DRGs or any subsequent change in reimbursement policy. All that we can expect is that we will evenutally refine our reimbursement techniques so that they will help to restrain the rate of increase in health care expenditures.

There is little prospect that in the foreseeable future government budgets at all levels, federal, state and local, will be freed from the intense pressures exerted by the continuing demands for more public dollars to pay for the health care of the elderly and the needy and to help maintain a strong infrastructure for medical education and research. Significant relief for governments would require a drastic turnabout in public attitudes such as an indifference to the consequences of cutbacks for the well-being of the elderly and the poor and a lack of concern by the body politic for maintaining U.S. medicine in a leadership role. Neither is likely to happen.

Moreover, it is unlikely that the broad health care insurance which most workers now receive from their employers will be drastically cut back. At most, we can expect more of what is now going on—some experimentation with trade-offs in the range and depth of coverage, copayments, and incentives for more economical use of benefits.

These cautionary observations about the slow pace of change in the years ahead may be read by some as a forecast of policy failure because it will leave us with many of the same problems that we have been unable to solve during the past decade. But there is an alternative interpretation: if this forecast is proved correct, it means that the generally high level of care available to most Americans will continue; the elderly and the poor will continue to have access to the system; financing will remain a constant problem, but enough money will continue to be forthcoming so that innovation will continue. In an imperfect world, such an outcome must be judged satisfactory if not ideal.

10

The Changing Health Care System

There are two ways of reading the tumultuous events that occurred on the health care front in New York City between 1964 and 1984. The first emphasizes the explosive rise in annual outlays, approximately $9 billion in inflation-free dollars, or almost threefold on a per capita basis. We have set out in Chapter 8 the principal effects of this much enlarged spending and have pinpointed the chief beneficiaries of these outlays among both patients and providers of health services.

There is a second way of assessing this tumultuous period and that is to note that despite the much enlarged inflow of dollars, the underlying structure of health care delivery in the City remained largely intact. To oversimplify: most physicians continued to treat patients on a fee-for-service basis in private offices where they practiced individually or in association with one or more colleagues. The large voluntary hospitals continued to be the dominant providers of inpatient care for the majority of citizens, with the municipal hospitals attending to large numbers of the poor.

In 1984 as in 1964, the City could count six medical schools located within its borders, although in the interim New York Medical College had relocated to suburban Westchester County and the Mt. Sinai School of Medicine of the City University of New York had opened its doors to students in 1968. The City's academic health centers continued to be in the forefront of both medical research and undergraduate and graduate medical education.

There is a strong probability that in the next decade to decade and a half, which will take us to the end of the century, we will witness the play upon the U.S. health care system of powerful forces stemming from changes in financing, market structures, human resources, and citizen behavior. While we cannot identify all of the forces much less calculate their outcome precisely, we should be able to delineate the broad interactions between these macro trends and the evolving health care structure in New York City. We will make the attempt; history will judge the accuracy of our forecasts.

To set the stage for this exercise in projection, we will list the more important national trends that are sufficiently established in 1985 to assure their future momentum:

- The accelerated attempts by all levels of government, employers, labor, and the citizenry at large to constrain the rate of increase in outlays for health care.
- The continuing large increases in the number of physicians entering the profession which many experts believe presage a supply of several types of specialists considerably in excess of the demand for their services.
- The emergence of a number of new systems for the financing and provision of health care, such as preferred provider organizations (PPOs), health maintenance organizations (HMOs) and their variants, walk-in clinics, hospitals specializing in the treatment of a single condition, and still other innovative forms.
- Major efforts to find alternatives to nursing homes for the increasing numbers of the frail elderly, many of whom find institutionalization expensive and undesirable.
- Intensified efforts by the federal and state governments through regulatory changes to alter market incentives and rewards with the aim of reducing tax outlays for health care and of simultaneously making the entire system less costly.
- Continuing pressure from the public for more and better health care services, universally accessible (the poor included), with a strong preference for prepayment over out-of-pocket financing.

The voluntary hospitals, and in particular the large teaching affiliates of the six academic health centers, are the driving force of the health care delivery system in New York City. Their relative importance has increased in recent decades as many smaller proprietary and voluntary hospitals have closed; as the municipal hospital system has contracted and depended for professional staffing on contractual relations with affiliates in the voluntary sector; and as the large voluntary institutions have become responsible for a growing proportion of hospital-based ambulatory care in the City. One revealing clue to the dominance of the major teaching hospitals has been their consistently high rate of occupancy—in the 90 percent range—during recent years.

The critical question is how these dominant institutions are likely to fare in the years ahead in the face of the diagnosis-related groups (DRGs), all-payer systems, the pressure for more treatment in ambulatory settings, cost increases stemming from large capital expenditures, changes in referral patterns, and still other forces that may emerge.

The applications of the major academic health centers for certificates of need to rehabilitate and modernize their aging facilities reflect their strong conviction that they will continue to operate in the future much as they have in the past. Without exception, their original proposals to Albany were predicated upon the maintenance of their present capacity with its strong bias in favor of inpatient services. Operating at the 90 percent occupancy level, they saw no reason to scale back the number of their beds.

Occupancy, as a criterion, is conditioned, however, upon the maintenance of adequate revenue flows to cover expenditures incurred for the given level of operations (with some surplus for innovation and improvements) if the institution is to retain solvency. The hospitals' planners may have given insufficient consideration to the powerful influences upon payers at present to depart from cost reimbursement and to constrain, if not eliminate, the opportunity for hospitals to cross-subsidize their operations by charging certain patients more thus compensating for others who pay less. The action of the Congress in 1983 to mandate prospective rate-setting based on DRGs for reimbursement by Medicare and the distinct possibility that all payers may sooner or later adopt the same approach present a major financial threat to the voluntary hospitals in New York City.

The first and overriding contributory factor is the excessive length of stay in New York City hospitals, the highest in the country, which is approximately 40 percent above that of comparable large urban hospitals in California. Since the regional and national reimbursement rates for DRGs will be determined in large measure by the average length of stay, New York City hospitals face the serious challenge of moving closer to the national norm, preferably below the norm.

Inasmuch as average length of stay has been steadily decreasing in New York City, particularly in the municipal system, there is some question about the remaining potential in this direction. To the extent, however, that the hospitals will succeed in achieving further reductions—and the pressure to do so will be severe—their bed requirements will moderate, probably substantially.

Strong reinforcement will come from the pressures that are building up from many sources to shift a greater volume of care from inpatient to ambulatory settings. In fact, many specialists believe that there are clear gains to the patient from such a shift and they are taking the lead to expand the practice of ambulatory surgery as well as of complex diagnostic and therapeutic procedures. Payers are introducing economic incentives to accomplish the same end by agreeing to cover all of the costs for ambulatory procedures but only part of the costs when the same procedures are performed in an inpatient setting.

Other factors that are likely to moderate the use of inpatient facilities are the expansion of enrollments in various prepaid delivery systems which are associated with much reduced hospital admission rates; the probability that Medicare beneficiaries will have to pay more out of pocket for inpatient care which would tend to reduce their level of demand; and the intensified competition between the increased supply of physicians and hospitals which will depress inpatient admissions. Further, as more and more competent physicians locate their practice in the suburbs, the number of referrals to the large teaching hospitals in the city will continue to decline. Finally, the increase of $100 or more in per diem rates to cover the costs of new construction will add one more hurdle to maintaining high occupancy rates in the major teaching hospitals in a period of fiscal constraint.

The more upbeat counterview about the future of the voluntary hospitals in New York City would stress that they are currently operating on an all-payer, non-DRG system, and may continue to do so in the future; that the rich pool of specialist talent in New York City is likely to continue to draw sufficient numbers of patients from beyond the City's limits to keep occupancy rates high; that the above-average number of elderly among the City's population with their differentially higher admission rates will also contribute to the maintenance of high occupancy; and that the training of large numbers of residents, which will surely continue, also contributes to the greater use of hospital facilities.

No matter how the occupancy issue resolves itself, it is difficult to foresee any circumstances in which the principal teaching affiliate of each of the academic health centers will not continue to be the institution of choice for many patients in and out of the city. More problematic is the future of selected independent voluntary hospitals that have large indigent patient rolls, and are in need of capital renovation. We know from the recent past that not all of these institutions have survived and if the financial environment should tighten, as we must anticipate, several other large voluntary hospitals may be at risk.

The major municipal hospitals—Bellevue, Harlem, North Central Bronx (NCB), Bronx Municipal Hospital Center (BMHC), Kings County, and Elmhurst—are in some cases so intricately intertwined with the operations of the several academic health centers—Downstate, New York University, Columbia-Presbyterian, Mt. Sinai, and Einstein—and are so critical to the delivery of health care to large concentrations of low-income groups that it is difficult to foresee the imminent or even ultimate closure of any of them. Their political-economic importance for the City's minority constituencies exercises an all but irresistible constraint upon their elimination. As one senior government official observed of the politically traumatic termination of Sydenham Hospital, a small, inefficient facility of admittedly low quality, "This is the last hospital closure that I ever intend to be involved in and I doubt whether the city will soon attempt any others."

Since the occupancy rates in municipal hospitals have been in the 80 percent range, the major opportunity for the system to tighten its operation is to cut back its authorized capacity and to orient its capital plans to a modernized but smaller plant with expanded ambulatory care facilities when funds become available. These are the guidelines for Kings County Hospital, which is among the first scheduled for reconstruction.

The last two decades have witnessed several conflicting trends with respect to the provision of ambulatory care. On the one hand, the dearth and ultimate disappearance of private practitioners in neighborhoods which have been abandoned by the middle class has resulted in the dependence of their present residents, the poor, on the local hospital for ambulatory care. A counter-development was the establishment and expansion of community health centers which provide a substitute for the vanishing private practitioner other than the hospital emergency room. A second substitute was the development of for-profit practice groups oriented to the Medicaid population. In terms of scale, hospital-based ambulatory care represented by far the largest of the three approaches.

Although New York City has one of the oldest and largest of all prepaid health care systems in the country—the Health Insurance Plan (HIP)—it has not demonstrated much capacity for growth in recent decades. As of 1983, the heart of its membership of 867,000 consists of municipal employees and the members of selected trade unions. The City has not been an encouraging environment up till now for the establishment and growth of new delivery systems. Early in 1974 Connecticut General established an HMO in Brooklyn which failed to attract the minimal necessary enrollment, lost a considerable sum, and was accordingly short-lived. Blue Cross/Blue Shield has also sought to stimulate HMO development, but thus far its efforts have met with only limited success. Its own effort, the Blue Cross/Blue Shield of Greater New York HMO, has a membership of 52,000.

What is responsible for the desultory growth of HMOs and the resistance of the City to new delivery systems? The explanation may be found in the preference of middle- and upper-income persons to select their own physicians; the preference of most physicians for fee-for-service or hospital-based practice; the disinclination of major hospitals to provide back-up arrangements; and the difficulties of constraining HMO staff from engaging in private practice on the side. Probably the most important determinant is the inability to identify sites within the City accessible to a critical mass of younger middle-class families who would be the natural constituency of an HMO. This population is now diffused throughout the suburban counties.

If one shifts focus from the middle class to the poor, one finds that they too have been hard to organize around a prepaid practice plan. One interesting experiment has been under way at Metropolitan: Montefiore has explored the potential of a prepaid plan in the South Bronx; and Governor Cuomo is committed to initiating demonstration projects among the Medicaid population. A first effort undertaken conjointly with the mayor in East Harlem met resistance from the local population and from state and local legislators over the issue of "lock-ins" and the abrogation of "freedom of choice" for the poor.

In its 1984 spring legislative session New York State took two actions with respect to ambulatory care: it raised the reimbursement rate for an emergency room visit to voluntary hospitals from $60 to $70 and it increased the schedule of physicians' fees for an office visit for Medicaid patients by 30 percent. It is questionable, however, that these actions of the legislature and the governor's expressed interest in stimulating enrollment of Medicaid patients in prepaid plans will effect major alterations in the existing patterns of ambulatory care during the next decade. Most middle-class residents will continue to seek care from private practitioners; most poor persons will continue to rely on the ambulatory facilities of neighborhood hospitals and to a lesser degree on community health centers, fee-for-service practitioner groups, and a small number of slow-growing prepaid practice organizations.

Other developments, however, may alter the foregoing. The combination of Medicare fiscal reforms which substantially increased copayments by users and which made a voucher system a more attractive incentive to prepaid plans to enroll the elderly, could result in the accelerated growth of prepayment groups. One must also allow for the possibility that some hospitals will expand the range of their market penetration by moving to develop new financing and delivery arrangements that will include the provision of ambulatory care services on a prepaid or fee-for-service basis or a combination of both. Moreover, some primary care services could be delivered at off-hospital sites, that is in satellite clinics or by arrangement with designated groups of physicians practicing in the community.

There is no question that for-profit corporations specializing in ambulatory care—walk-in clinics, emergi-centers, surgi-centers—have extended beyond their initial centers of growth in the South and the

West to open facilities in the Midwest, and are exploring opportunities in the Northeast which till now has been an unfriendly market. The question that we face is whether the combination of the particular health care market in New York City and the strong regulatory structure in Albany will make it unlikely, if not impossible, for corporate medicine to establish a presence in New York City. While it is difficult to foresee a strong movement towards the establishment in New York City of for-profit ambulatory facilities in the decade ahead, the prospect cannot be totally ruled out. In this connection it is well to recall that for-profit nursing homes were able to grow rapidly in the New York City area at the same time that many proprietary hospitals were forced to close their doors.

In addition to the growth of proprietary nursing home beds, the last decades have seen the expansion of nonprofit nursing home capacity; a substantial government effort to care for Medicaid patients in their own homes; and recent experimental programs (the "Nursing Home Without Walls" championed by Senator Tarky Lombardi is an example) that provide community-based services aimed at reducing prospective admissions of middle-class and Medicaid patients to nursing homes.

Despite widespread belief to the contrary, New York City and the United States will not experience over the next ten to fifteen years any substantial increase in the number of the elderly and particularly the frail elderly, that is persons over 85. The large demographic shifts will only occur after the year 2010 when the baby boom generation reaches retirement age. Nonetheless the steady upward drift in the number of elderly will keep the question of how best to respond to their health and related needs in the foreground.

Responding to expenditures of over $400 million annually by New York City for care of Medicaid beneficiaries remaining in their own homes, the State legislature acted to limit the size of the program by capping the financial contribution of the State. With an average of about fifty hours per week of home care aides' services, the cost of preventing admissions to nursing homes comes high, about $15,000 per person per year net of rent, food, and utilities.

To assess the prospect of a significant shift to home care, several interconnected questions need to be sorted out. As spokespeople for the elderly have stressed, other things being equal, most elderly prefer to remain at home rather than seek admission to a nursing home. But often, complicating factors of family, health, and money intervene. It is much easier for a frail elderly person to remain at home if there are family members living in the same household or close by. The extent to which the homebound need assistance is a critical variable. One of the largest for-profit home health agencies has calculated that the breakpoint is around four hours of assistance five days a week, or approximately twenty hours of externally provided care. Family or friends are expected to provide assistance over the weekend. Then there is the question of money. Is the elderly person using his own funds or does he rely on public dollars? The range and quality of community services for the homebound and the availability of congregate housing are also important considerations.

Other factors that will influence the patterns of health care for the elderly in the remaining years of this century will be the extension of DRG-based reimbursement which will tend to shorten hospital stays and necessitate more extensive follow-up care at home for discharged patients; the extent to which the Medicare voucher gains acceptance and encourages large-scale enrollment of the elderly in HMOs and similar prepaid groups; improvements in medical technology and equipment that will ease the problems of caring for the severely disabled at home; and changing values among the elderly themselves that will affect decisions on heroic treatment and terminal care.

A middle of the road forecast which does not pretend to assess definitively all of the foregoing factors suggests that there is likely to be a relative shift from inpatient to ambulatory and home care treatment settings; that the expansion of hospices will continue; that if and when acute care hospitals find themselves with excess capacity, they will be likely to convert some of their beds to rehabilitation and the care of the elderly; that more people will prefer to die at home to avoid being subjected to extreme forms of medical or surgical intervention; and that there will remain substantial pressures on nursing home capacity for a variety of reasons, including the inability of many of the frail elderly to manage on their own.

The last forecast would, of course, be modified if medical research found techniques to slow if not reverse senile dementia and to strengthen bladder and bowel control among the elderly. It is unlikely that these breakthroughs will be realized within a single decade, but if they were, admissions to nursing homes would stabilize and might even decline.

So far we have concentrated on the changes that the different settings within which health care has been provided—hospitals, physicians offices and clinics, nursing homes, and home care—are likely to undergo in response to the preferences of patients, the expenditures of financers, or alterations in the ways in which physicians and other health care providers shape their careers and their work.

We must now shift our focus to another critical dimension of the health care sector in New York City, that is its role in the education and training of physicians both at the undergraduate and graduate level—a major function of the City's six academic health centers and their affiliated teaching hospitals. This educational function is directly and intimately linked to the provision of hospital and ambulatory care for a significant proportion of the City's residents and plays a dominant role in the care provided the low-income population by the municipal hospitals, the Veterans Administration hospitals, and the inpatient and ambulatory services of the voluntary hospitals.

It has been observed that the academic health centers perform a disproportionate amount of the nation's residency training, roughly four times the City's share relative to its population. To a lesser degree, they also educate a disproportionate number of undergraduate medical students, more than double New York's percentage of population. The vast scale of undergraduate and graduate instruction and training carried on in New York City requires us to consider the factors on the local, state, and national scenes that are likely to affect this particular dimension of the health care sector.

It is important to note that the assumption prevailing throughout the first three post–World War II decades—that the nation, New York State, and New York City would all profit from the training of an increased number of physicians—is no longer conventional wisdom. The Report of the Graduate Medical Educational National Advisory Committee (GMENAC), published in 1980, presented an impressive body of data and analysis that questioned the validity of the perception of a continuing physician shortage. Admittedly, the leadership of U.S. medicine did not accept, surely not initially, the alternative finding of a prospective surplus. Despite the fact that New York City and New York State ranked among the highest in their ratios of physicians to population, their political and professional leadership were also counted among the skeptics. The State Board of Regents has persistently maintained that since many rural and low-income urban areas lack the number of private practitioners required to provide adequate care to their residents, a policy of selective expansion in the training of physicians is necessary, surely desirable. Other state agencies, sensitive to the relatively small numbers of minorities in the medical profession and in the educational pipeline, have also looked to an expansionary policy to correct these imbalances.

New York State, and in particular the New York metropolitan region, have also spawned a vociferous citizen lobby on behalf of state and federal action to facilitate the receipt of a medical education abroad by their children who failed to gain admission to U.S. medical schools despite the doubling of their capacity.

The borough of Queens has agitated for many years to become the site of a medical school, its leaders emphasizing repeatedly that Manhattan, Bronx, and Brooklyn all contain at least one. In 1984 the State Legislature finally transferred a modest sum, about $1.5 million, from the budget of the State University to that of the City University to encourage the latter to move ahead on planning for a medical school in Queens linked to the City University. Whether this authorization of funds will in fact bring the school into existence remains uncertain in the face of the State's disinclination to provide the bulk of the required monies; the determination of City College (located in Manhattan) not to relinquish the Sophie Davis School which provides preclinical training for many minority students pursuing a medical education; and the preference of Downstate Medical Center to expand its linkages to its affiliates in Brooklyn rather than to expand to a Queens clinical campus.

Several other facts bearing on undergraduate enrollment should be noted. SUNY-Downstate Medical School which has the largest student body of any of the six schools in the City has been advised by the accreditation authorities that it must strengthen its curriculum. The State of New York has been unwilling to invest sizable new funds to reinforce Downstate and it has also reached the limit of what it is willing to invest in Stony Brook which remains a small school, far below original projections.

The State Health Commissioner also has recently acted to tighten the conditions under which U.S. citizens who study medicine in foreign schools may receive clerkships and staff appointments in hospitals in New York State which particularly affects New York City facilities.

In light of these conflicting forces and trends a cautionary view would suggest that the Queens medical school will continue to have a difficult gestation. At the same time it is unlikely that there will be any cutback in the present level of undergraduate medical enrollment in the near term. A few years ago it was rumored that Albany would favor the elimination, through merger or relocation, of one of the private medical schools in New York City but of late that has not been heard. And unless the State's budgetary condition were to worsen appreciably, it would appear that Bundy money—state capitation aid to private institutions for the education of health care professionals—is likely to continue.

The outlook for residency training is more complex. There are several critical interrelated aspects to the scale and scope of residency training. To begin with, much of the renown of the major academic health centers in New York City is directly linked to their long-term leadership in the field of graduate medical education. Some years ago when the State authorities, in an effort to reduce Medicaid reimbursement levels, placed a ceiling on the number of residents that the large teaching hospitals could include in their cost base for reimbursement, several of the leaders acted jointly to challenge this action in the courts and won their case with the argument that the State officials had exceeded their authority in seeking to set an educational quota for these institutions.

The post–World War II decades have witnessed a shift in the staffing of the major teaching hospitals and this, in turn, has effected basic changes in the manner in which different groups of patients are treated. The major teaching hospitals, which previously depended on attending physicians, are now dominated by full-time senior staff who admit and oversee the treatment of most private patients. However, they rely increasingly on residents and fellows to provide much of the routine care, from pre-operative testing to post-operative support services.

There is no way to draw a sharp demarcation between the educational experiences that the house staff is exposed to and the service functions that they perform. Most informed observers believe that surely after the first year, and often even during the first year, the patient service provided by house staff more than justifies the salaries that they are paid and that their "pure" educational activities consume only a small proportion of their lengthy daily and weekly schedules.

The house staff is also responsible for much or most of the outpatient care provided in the emergency room and in the clinics and for inpatients who do not have a private physician at the time of admission, although a member of the full-time staff may formally assume responsibility to permit the hospital to claim reimbursement under Medicare B (professional services) as well as under Medicare A (hospitalization).

In comparison with the major voluntary teaching hospitals, the residents' role in patient care is far greater in the municipal and the VA hospitals with which most teaching hospitals are affiliated. Since the early 1960s, when the affiliation program was introduced, the municipal hospitals have depended overwhelmingly on residents and fellows for the bulk of the ambulatory and inpatient care that they provide. True, the contracting teaching affiliate provides supervisory staff to assure that the prescribed diagnostic and therapeutic procedures are appropriate and are competently performed, but the great bulk of the care is provided by residents and the scope and quality of their supervision differs considerably among contractors and even among divisions and clinical departments under the control of the same contractor.

The relationship between the medical centers and the Veterans Administration hospitals has been relatively satisfactory these many years, largely as a result of the availability of substantial funding which enabled the VA hospitals to maintain good support services as well as to pursue an impressive volume of in-house research and to support broad-based educational programs. More recently, funding from Washington has tightened and the VA hospitals are under increasing pressure to redirect their resources to expanding ambulatory care with corresponding economies in inpatient services that are the foundation for their cooperative residency programs. Research funding has also been cut back.

The primary affiliations of the academic health centers in New York City, however, have been with the much larger municipal hospital system. Three of the six medical schools—Downstate, New York University, and Einstein—depend in the first instance on a municipal hospital for most of their undergraduate and graduate clinical teaching. Mt. Sinai and Columbia also are affiliated with municipal hospitals although these are less critical to their total teaching function. Only Cornell is without such an affiliation.

There have been and continue to be tensions between the contractors and the affiliates since the onset of the program in the early 1960s. The major difficulties have centered around deficiencies in the support services provided by the municipal hospitals, ranging from diagnostic equipment to nursing care. For its part, the City has repeatedly remonstrated with the contractors that they have been more concerned with providing acceptable training for their residents than addressing the priority needs of the patients who seek care in the municipal hospitals and assigning staff to meet these needs. A quarter of a century after the inauguration of the affiliation program the conflicting interests of the two parties continue, with each round of negotiations seeking to narrow the gap.

It is unlikely that either party is in a position to withdraw from the contract, at least in the near term. If a radical reduction should occur in the number of inpatient days, conceivably the municipal hospitals could—in light of the easing of the physician market—recruit and retain an increasing number of full-time staff and thereby reduce their dependency on contractual relations. But it is difficult to see how they could operate without a large complement of residents and how these trainees could be attracted other than with the support of a major academic health center. Accordingly, the present uneasy alliance between the medical centers and the Health and Hospitals Corporation is likely to persist for some years to come.

The third dimension that will determine the future scale of residency training relates to the overarching issue of financing. It seems incredible, but is nonetheless a fact, that the vast expansion of graduate medical education during the past decades has come about in the absence of a generic financing mechanism. Aside from the mixed transaction by which residents provide services with relatively modest pay in return for educational and training opportunities, most other

costs incidental to their training have been covered by reimbursements for patient care. Insurance and government have accepted the
costs of operating educational programs as a legitimate item in patient
reimbursement.

Recently, challenges to this practice have begun to mount. The most
important thus far has been the unanimous recommendation of the
Social Security Advisory Council that a funding mechanism other
than Medicare should be developed to support residency training. In
initiating DRGs, Congress bypassed this issue by providing a pass-
through for educational costs but the Secretary of the Department of
Health and Human Services was directed to study this problem and
come forward with specific recommendations as to the preferred ways
of reimbursing hospitals for the additional costs of training residents.

The current pass-through provisions for DRGs which take into
account not only direct educational outlays but also higher ancillary
costs referable to increased length of stay and greater intensity of
care—both presumptively linked with residency training—have
proved favorable to the academic health centers, but it is unlikely that
Congress will continue them beyond the next few years. It remains
unclear, however, what alternative approach will be acceptable to the
Congress, the states, and the private sector, each of which currently
helps to underwrite graduate medical education and each of which
will be under pressure to continue to support in one way or another
this essential activity on which the medical care of the future is
dependent.

The financing question is linked to the growing concern of many
specialty societies about the number of residents who should be
trained; the number of hospitals that may for economic or other
reasons opt to reduce or terminate their training activities; and national and regional ratios of the number of U.S. medical graduates to
the number of training slots. We are approaching a position where,
for the first time, the two are in approximate balance which means
that any substantial reduction of the training programs could result in
the failure of some graduates to gain acceptance to an approved
program.

The outlook for residency training in New York City will be influ-
enced by the interactions among several factors: the large scale of the
current programs; the dependence of the public hospitals (and also
the voluntary hospitals) for the provision of patient care on the
availability of large numbers of residents; the uncertainty of future
financing from public and private sources for the higher hospital costs
associated with residency training; and the pressures arising within
various specialty societies to scale back training programs. We cannot
make even an educated guess as to the interactive effects of these

discrete forces other than that on balance they point to a reduction over time in the scale and scope of residency training by the hospitals of New York City. If the payers for hospital care were to take radical action to decrease or eliminate their contributions for such training, an unlikely but not impossible step, and if no satisfactory alternative were devised, the reduction could be substantial. The more likely eventuality, however, will be modest cutbacks that over time could be absorbed without major threat to the current provision of patient care or the training of tomorrow's physicians.

We are now approaching the end of the scenario for the future. The one remaining critical issue to be discussed is the role of state regulation. Currently, and for some time in the past, the State of New York has exercised substantial influence and control over hospital reimbursements, capital improvements, and the regional distribution of services; most recently it has introduced an all-payer system to distribute the costs of care for the uninsured. There is no reason to believe that the State will withdraw from any of these activities and there is reason to postulate that it will assume an even more prominent role in shaping the structure of the health care system in New York City and the remainder of the State. There are also indications from Washington that point to a growing preference by the federal government to devolve more responsibility for the control of future outlays for health care onto the states. If we assume that such a policy will gain momentum—and this seems likely, because of the difficulties of establishing national norms for the various states whose systems operate under quite different environmental conditions—we must anticipate a more active role for State officials in the reshaping of the City's health care system. A clue to the nature and intensity of the State's involvement is found in the pressure that it is exerting in response to the certificate of need (CON) applications filed by the academic health centers. To both Presbyterian Hospital and Mt. Sinai, the Commissioner of Health has indicated that approval was contingent upon a trade: the more responsibility these institutions were willing to undertake to assist their neighboring communities—in the case of Presbyterian, the establishment of a new community hospital at the northern tip of Manhattan, and in the case of Mt. Sinai supporting North General Hospital in Harlem—the better their prospects for receiving approval. Similarly, Cornell, which is also seeking CON approval, has been urged to extend its existent ties with Jamaica Hospital in Queens.

The State has also indicated that it plans to step up its role in determining the location of costly new services (such as Nuclear Magnetic Resonators) with the aim of avoiding unnecessary, costly overcapacity and underutilization.

The legislature acted recently to strengthen the Health Services Agencies, the planning bodies throughout the state, to get their input as to how finite capital funds should be allocated within the several regions so that priority needs should be met equitably. The federal government will act shortly on the capital pass-through in the determination of Medicare reimbursement rates; thereafter the states are likely to have a clearer view of their future scope for action. But no matter what actions Congress takes regarding the capital pass-through, it is well-nigh certain that the State of New York will continue to play a major role in shaping the directions of future hospital investments.

The remaining important arena for present and potential state action relates to all-party payer arrangements to meet the costs of non-reimbursed care for the indigent. New York State has long been sensitive to this issue and as early as 1970 enacted the Ghetto Medicine Program which made special grants to help urban hospitals increase services to the inner-city populations. In 1982 it received a waiver from the Department of Health and Human Services (HHS) of standard Medicare reimbursement provisions that permitted the institution of an all-payer system. This system imposes a levy on all hospitals to be contributed to a pool for distribution to those institutions that furnish large amounts of unrequited care.

It is doubtful whether HHS will extend the limited number of waivers it has authorized which have permitted New York and several other states to operate all-payer systems, but in light of the progressive devolution of control to the states, it is reasonable to assume that Albany will maintain the present system or substitute another that will socialize at least in part the expenditures that hospitals incur in treating large numbers of the uninsured poor.

Given the many uncertainties that exist, it would be presumptuous to venture an outline of the future shape of the health care system in New York City viewed through a prism focused on the years 1990—2000. However some synthesis of the many discrete trends and possibilities that have been identified would be desirable if only to orient the reader to the future. We will make the attempt, reemphasizing that the scenario contains many problematic factors; the margin of uncertainty is heightened when allowance is made for the interaction among the major elements. Despite these caveats, the effort may be justified.

- The relative role of hospital care within the health care system will decline in favor of greater reliance on ambulatory services, home care, and nursing home and hospice care.
- The major voluntary hospitals in New York City face a serious

financial threat from the DRG approach because of their excessive lengths of stay. Even if the DRG approach should be radically modified or replaced, hospitals whose length of stay and
per diem costs far exceed the average are certain to be under
financial stress in a period of continuing price pressure.

- The combination of these two developments is likely to produce
within the next five years, and surely within the next ten years, a
shift from high occupancy rates to an excess of beds in most of
the large hospitals.
- It is unlikely that the municipal hospital system which experienced a substantial contraction in the preceding two decades
will shrink further through major closures in the period ahead.
However, it is likely to reduce its total inpatient bed capacity as
part of its capital rehabilitation program.
- The State of New York will continue to discourage the expansion of nursing home capacity and will maintain a ceiling on the
elaboration by New York City of its home care program because
of the serious implications of further expansion for state expenditures. The thrust of the State (as well as of the federal
government and the voluntary sector) will be to strengthen
support efforts that will enable more of the frail elderly to be
cared for in their own homes and communities. However, these
constraining attempts may conflict with the reality of an expanded cohort of feeble elderly who will require institutional
care, particularly if the restrictions on new capacity are maintained for the next five to ten years.
- The uncertainties regarding the future financing of graduate
medical education point to prospective adjustments in the very
large training programs in New York City, adjustments that are
likely to result in reductions in training and in some cooperative
arrangements among the major academic health centers for the
conduct of high cost, low-volume subspecialty programs. Such
cooperative undertakings are not easy to negotiate and imple-
ment but they may be preferable to the complete elimination of
selected programs. These developments are more likely if individual specialty societies take the lead to cut back training programs and if the State throws its weight behind reductions in
the hope of moderating costs.

The more problematic issues involve the future of undergraduate
enrollments, methods of financing the care of the poor, and the
growth of new forms of health care delivery. We noted earlier that
despite the long-time enthusiasm of Queens residents for a medical
school within their borough and the recent transfer of State funds to

the City University budget for planning purposes, serious questions remain about the feasibility of this long-term objective. The minimum funding is simply not there nor is it in sight; the medical establishment is equivocal about the addition of another school; the most suitable hospital to serve as a clinical facility for the school would be Long Island Jewish Medical Center and it is questionable whether the Jewish voluntary community in New York City which already supports two medical schools—Einstein and Mt. Sinai—is prepared to divert philanthropic funds to the development of another. Finally the present sponsor (City College) of the Sophie Davis preclinical medical program is opposed to its transfer to Queens. While the location of the preclinical program in proximity to the newly organized clinical campus is not a necessary condition for the operation of a Queens medical school, there has been pressure for it. It does not follow that despite these formidable obstacles the new school will not be established, but it would require an unusually favorable concatenation of circumstances to speed its opening.

In fact, a trend to reduce undergraduate enrollments in the existing schools is not beyond the realm of possibility. New York University has already taken a small step in that direction. In a state that has long followed an expansionary policy such a reduction will not be easy to effect but it cannot be ruled out. If physicians in private practice experienced a serious continuing loss in real income, they might persuade the legislature that cutbacks in the publicly supported schools would be desirable. This recommendation has been made to Downstate by the accrediting authority. The State could also cut back, even if it does not totally eliminate, capitation support for the private schools.

Since the major teaching hospitals and selected community hospitals provide a considerable amount of care to uninsured patients, and since most of them do not have the revenues to cover the deficits that they incur thereby, the State will confront the necessity of finding an alternative to the current all-payer system which it has initiated by means of a Medicare waiver from the Department of HHS. If, as is likely, the federal waiver is terminated, the State will probably continue the all-payer system on its own initiative.

Perhaps the most problematic of future developments is the extent to which new forms of health care delivery will emerge and succeed. HMOs do not appear to be poised for rapid growth but the State, in cooperation with the City, may force the issue as regards Medicaid recipients. If the federal voucher for Medicare is made more attractive both to the beneficiaries and to the providers, this will stimulate the growth of HMOs and other types of prepayment plans.

It is difficult to discern whether, on what scale, and how quickly the large teaching hospitals are likely to expand the scale and scope of their activities, from new ambulatory care services for paying patients to rehabilitation and hospice care. Their long experience with high occupancy rates will probably deter serious efforts at innovation.

Even more difficult to assess is whether and in which areas new for-profit medical enterprises will seek to enter the New York City market. The proprietary chains have given the City a wide berth in years past because they saw little opportunity for profits in an environment in which the State exercises tight control over reimbursement, licensing, and other facets of the system. Another deterrent is the prohibition by State law of the absentee ownership of health facilities. Since the State is likely to maintain tight control via CON, licensing, as well as reimbursement rate-setting, the odds are that a decade hence the for-profit institutions will still have only a marginal role in New York City.

The foregoing scenario relates primarily to process. The major issue is whether the health care system currently in place will perform as well or better both in meeting the health needs of the population and in encouraging the continued vitality of the system through its contributions to education and research. To comment on the latter issue first, it is difficult to foresee a serious weakening in the major academic health centers. All but Downstate have sizable endowments, are linked to strong universities, and are closely affiliated with major voluntary hospitals. For its part, Downstate will probably continue to command substantial State and City resources.

The answer to the first question as to the scale and quality of health care services that will be available to the citizenry as the century draws to a close also must be basically upbeat. There is no reason to believe that the combination of the large voluntary institutions, reinforced by the extensive municipal hospital system should not be able to provide in the future, as they do at present and have in the past, a superior level of care to the more affluent population and an acceptable level to the poor and the near poor. They should be able to meet this challenge in the face of a more constrained inflow of funds and necessary modifications in the locus of care. Only a collapse of leadership among the medical profession, the voluntary community, and City and State politicians—a highly unlikely eventuality—would place the system at serious risk. To the extent that the three groups deepen their understanding of the dynamics of change and develop more effective cooperation, the quality of care available to all should be improved.

Notes

Chapter 2

[1] Nora Piore, Purlaine Lieberman, and James Linnane, "Public Expenditures and Private Control? Health Care Dilemmas in New York City," *Milbank Memorial Fund Quarterly/Health and Society,* Winter 1977, pp. 79–116.

[2] Eli Ginzberg and Matthew P. Drennan, *A Commonwealth Fund Paper: The Health Sector—Its Significance for the Economy of New York City* (New York: The Commonwealth Fund, 1985).

Chapter 3

[1] United Hospital Fund, *A Decade of Change in New York City* (New York: United Hospital Fund, February 1981).

[2] United Hospital Fund, *Hospital Manpower in New York City* (New York: United Hospital Fund, 1980).

Chapter 4

[1] Eli Ginzberg, *A Pattern for Hospital Care* (New York: Columbia University, 1949).

[2] Eli Ginzberg and Peter Rogatz, *Planning for Better Hospital Care* (New York: Columbia University, 1961).

Chapter 6

[1] State Health Manpower Policy Advisory Council, *Graduate Medical Education* (New York, February 1983).

[2] United Hospital Fund, *Foreign Medical Graduates in New York City* (New York: United Hospital Fund, 1978).

[3] New York State Department of Education, *Physician Manpower Survey 1980–1981,* April 1982.

[4] United Hospital Fund, *Hospital Manpower in New York City* (New York: United Hospital Fund, June 1980).

Index

Community Mental Health Board, 70
Community Mental Health Clinic, 48–49
Community orientation of hospitals, 62
Competitive market and health care, 134–35
Comprehensive Health Care Center, 64
Congregation of the Sisters of Charity, 46, 62
Connecticut General, 141
Conservation of Human Resources, 37
Conservation Project, 43
Consumer Price Index, inflation in, 111
Convalescent facilities, 42
Cornell University, 150
Cost of Living Council, 101–102
Cuomo, Mario, 142

Davis, Leon, 98–99, 101–103, 105, 109
Decade of Change in New York City Hospital Services, A, 32
Deinstitutionalization of mental patients, 118
Delafield Hospital, 102
Dental services, 17, 27
  public and private expenditures, 19–21, 75
Department of Health, 65, 70, 74
  programs operated by, 66
Department of Health and Human Services, 149, 151, 153
Department of Hospitals, 57
Department of Human Resources, 114
Department of Mental Hygiene, 70
Department of Welfare, 70
Dewey, Thomas, 54
Diagnosis-related group (DRG) system of reimbursement, 131, 139, 144, 149, 152
Disabled, medical care of, 2, 17
  Medicare and, 70
Downstate Medical Center, 31, 53, 90, 140, 146
Downstate Medical School, 65, 82, 146, 148, 153, 154
Downstate University Hospital, 87, 119–20
Drennan, Matthew, 15
Drug abuse, 73
Drug and Hospital Workers Union, Local 1199, 97–106, 109
Drugs, 17, 23
  cost reimbursement for, 27
  public and private expenditures, 19, 21
  Drugs and appliances, public sector contribution, 70–71, 75

Educational requirements for health care positions, 95
Einstein College Hospital, 59, 60–61, 63

Einstein Medical School, 53, 55, 65, 140, 148, 153
Elderly, increase in, 15, 143
Elderly, health care of, 2, 6, 9, 11–12, 17, 24–25, 30, 33, 70, 114–15
  ambulatory care, dependence on, 10
  home care of, 152
  hospital admissions of, 71–72, 140
  outreach care and, 48, 143–44
  poverty and, 8, 68
  reimbursement of health costs, 27
Elmhurst Hospital, 140
Emergency care, 33, 34
Emergency Financial Control Board, 104
Emergency room visits, 48, 50, 73
Entrepreneurship, public, 5, 64
Environmental factors in assessing health status, 113
Extended care services in hospitals, 60

Family Health Center, 64
Federal funding for health services, 73, 78, 129–30
Federation of Jewish Philanthropies, 4, 58
Feinstein, Barry, 98
Female hospital workers, 95
Flower Fifth Avenue, 119
FMGs. *See* Foreign medical graduates
Foner, Moe, 105
Fordham Hospital, 102
Foreign medical graduates, 26, 40, 74, 82–83, 90, 123
Full-time equivalent employees (FTE), 39

Gaus, Clifton R., 73
General care hospitals, 56, 62, 95
  decline in, 30–31
  discharges from, 33
  patient days, total, 42
  service divisions, 35
General practitioners, 30, 85, 116, 122–23
Ghetto Medicine Program, 151
Goodoff, Elliot, 105
Gotbaum, Victor, 100–102, 107, 109–10
Gouverneur Hospital, 102
Government contribution to health care, 132, 135
Government grants, loans, 62
Government reductions in health care outlays, 133
Government regulation of reimbursement, 131
Grace, William J., 47
Graduate medical education, 30, 36, 54, 60, 81–82, 152–53
  costs of, 87–88
  practice location and, 81

Senile patients, 118
Sickroom supplies, 23
Simon, William, 103
Skilled nursing facilities (SNF), 41–42
Skilled nursing services in hospitals, 35
Social Security Act, 31
　Title XIII, 11. *See also* Medicare
　Title XIX, 11. *See also* Medicaid
Social Security Advisory Council, 149
Social Security benefits, 68
Sophie Davis School, 146, 153
Southern Manhattan Dialysis Center, 53
Specialists, 7, 30, 54–55, 92, 116–17, 123, 140
　distribution of, 85, *86*
　income of, 91
Specialized hospitals, 36
Special services in hospitals, 38, 40, 39
　expenditures for, 37
　staff salary expenditures, 52
Spend-down provision for Medicaid eligibility, 27
Spofford Juvenile Detention Center, 64
St. Luke's-Roosevelt Hospital, 120
St. Vincent's Hospital and Medical Center, 4–5, 46–54, 62–63, 102, 120
State Department of Education, 84, 91
State Health Manpower Policy Advisory Council, 81
State hospitals, 39
Stony Brook Medical School, 146
Strikes, hospital, 86, 101–104, 101–105, 109
Suburbs, increase in hospitals in, 31
SUNY-Downstate Medical School. *See* Downstate Medical School
Supervisory physicians, 40, 60, 87, 90–91, 121–22, 147
Supplemental Medical Insurance (SMI), 17
Supplemental Security Income program (SSI), 118
Surgeons, income of, 91
Surgical specialties, 53
Sydenham Hospital, 102, 141

Teaching hospitals, 2, 7, 30, 31, 55, 62, 66, 81, 92, 115, 119–20, 138–39, 154
　medical progress and, 29
　salary expenses, 87
　voluntary, 5–6
Teamsters Union, Local 237, 97
Tertiary care services of hospitals, 53, 63
Third-party reimbursement, 4, 8, 50, 58, 127
　hospitals, effect on, 130–31
Thompson, Paul, 59
Trussell, Ray, 66
Tuberculosis services in hospitals, 35, 60
Turner, Doris, 105

Uninsured patients, 8, 153
　all-payer system for care of, 150–51
Unionization of health care workers, 6, 97–100. *See also specific unions*
Unions
　civil service, 104
　trade, 9
United Hospital Fund (UHF), 30, 32, 39, 73, 87, 88, 106, 120
University Hospital at Einstein Medical College, 119
US-FMGs, 90, 123

VA hospitals, 147–48
Valhalla Hospital, 80
Van Arsdale, Harry, 109
Veterans Administration, 70. *See also* VA hospitals
Village Nursing Home, 48
Visiting Nurse Service, 48
Voluntary hospitals, 3, 31–32, 46, 135, 137, 138–40
　ambulatory care, 73
　city reimbursement for patient care, 65
　collective bargaining, statutes re, 98
　diagnosis-related groups system of reimbursement and, 150–51
　employee increases, 39, 96, 106
　expenditures of, 23
　hospitalization insurance and, 108
　long-term care in, 41–42
　monetarization of, 69
　nonprofessional employees of, 8–9
　occupancy rate, 33
　outpatient visits, 33–34
　patient days, total, 32
　patients' choice of, 72
　poor, care of, 26, 132
　public sector contribution, 77
　residency training program in, 36
　role of, 10
　service divisions, 35–36
　types of, 119
　workers' earnings, *107*
　See also Teaching hospitals
Voluntary medical staff, 47
Volunteer physicians, 88, 122
Voucher system for health care delivery, 142

Wages, minimum weekly, 98, 100–102
Wagner, Robert, 98, 109
Ward care in hospitals, 46
Well-baby clinics, 65
Working poor, 25, 26, 68–69

Yeshiva University, 55